WHEN WAS IT
I DARED TO DREAM

The Journey of a Soul Incarnate

by
Barbara Lee Duffy

With John M. Flynn

WHEN WAS IT I DARED TO DREAM
The Journey of a Soul Incarnate
Published in America
by Tailgate Press.

Book design by John M. Flynn
Cover design by John M. Flynn with Kelsey Roy

Tailgatepress@gmail.com

ISBN-13: 978-0-692-97868-9

ISBN-10: 0-692-97868-2

Contents

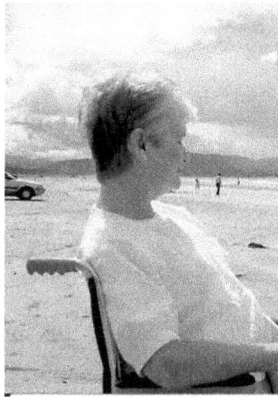

Who Am I

I am a friend I am a teacher
I am a counselor
I am a story teller
I am a woman.
I am a woman with a disability
I use a wheelchair
I ask for help
I work
I make love
I play
I care for my friends
I pray
I am fully grown up
Finally
and now in my prime
I have a story to tell
Straightforwardly for what it's worth...
The Journey of a Soul Incarnate.

This book is dedicated to the loving, caring person who created it—
Barbara Lee Duffy

Yes,

I am writing my story and I plan to strip my story bare of all that is not essential—all that is unnecessary—all that is not needed. So that what *is* needed, what *is* essential and necessary will stand out clearly visible, alive and passionate. So that my soul will have a vibrant essence—so that the divinity at the core of my being—the essential form, will fully emerge, as life itself.

Love,

Barbara

Preface

In the event that you don't know her, or only know of her, let me introduce my cousin, Barbara Lee Duffy, to you and explain how I got involved with her memoir. Barbara was born in 1939 and raised in an Irish Catholic family in Stoneham, Massachusetts. Those were the days before the Salk vaccine was available and Polio was running rampant among every level of American society. Barbara found out all about it at the age of ten, when on a steamy hot afternoon in July of 1949 she found herself in an iron lung at Children's Hospital in Boston, where her life was saved, restarted anew and altered for good. How much the same or different was it, you may ask, than any other child who had lost the use of most of his or her body parts and had to learn how to breathe again? The difference was that Barbara carried within her a great secret that other recipients of that debilitating disease were not privy to– a supreme secret she could not share with them because if she did, she was convinced the new world that was now keeping her together would crash and burn and they would despise her for including them. She could never tell them what caused their Polio without losing the vital focus necessary in keeping her alert and paying strict attention, so crucial to the continued existence of her new self.

Barbara and I were linked in a mystical/spiritual vortex from the days we were toddlers until and beyond the time she passed away on August 2, 2015. In deference to my ten years on the road, she used to say that she was like Emily Dickinson sitting in her yard clicking her knitting needles together, while I was out there on the road sweeping wavelike around the country, like Walt Whitman.

In the waning days of the year 2000 I was working on a novel and acting in local theaters. Barbara phoned and said that she had something important to discuss with me. I hurried over and found her on the sun-deck. She handed me four computer diskettes. She said that she hadn't yet organized it into book form and she needed my help with the formatting, editing and rewrites where necessary.

I must admit, I didn't exactly leap into it, but I did *look* into it, at first gingerly, until I read the following words and found myself knocked out cold.

"A child of ten, I was. A child of ten. Ordinary. With freckles. Wearing blue overalls and sneakers. Always set and ready for surprises! And oh yes, surprises did come. New people. A new script. A whole new way of being in

1

this world. I was ten one minute and ageless the next. I was standing tall and ready for anything one minute and the next minute I was paralyzed–unable to breathe, eat, roll over, pee or swallow my tears. My life began anew that day–anew in the big yellow tank–The Iron Lung–my cocoon. Finally, I was warm and safe and cared for."

From that moment on I was hooked. I should say totally involved and by the spring of 2013, I had finished working on most of her earlier pages and had about fifty more left to weave into it. She told me that we should classify this memoir as a joint work/collaboration because even though it was all about her and although she had periodically received some assistance from friends, it was mostly help in the form of opinion.

On Thanksgiving, I baked a turkey and brought it over to Barbara's, along with the pages I had worked on, while Barbara provided the hot dogs, apple juice and B&M brown-bread.

After we ate and went over the pages, she handed me another twenty-five sheets and said, "This is all I've got for now." We sat together on that pleasant Thanksgiving Day for hours. Being that it was only the two of us on such an important Holiday, we chuckled, because it looked as though we both had burnt a few bridges. We had. That was the last time I saw Barbara alive. At her Wake I mentioned to a few of her friends that I was working on her memoir. Had I known that my words were going to elicit such a plethora of icy responses, I would have kept my mouth shut. I think they were scared to death they might be in it. They were right. They are!!!

Barbara told me years before that she planned to publish her writings, so what she said next surprised me a little. "If I should pass on and we aren't done, I want you to put everything together and finish it. In other words, make a book out of it, because I have changed my mind and don't want it published until I'm gone. I have my reasons for that and you don't need to know them. But at this juncture in my life, I do know that you are the only one I can trust to do this right."

Since Barbara moved on to the next square, it has taken me two years more to complete her story as she had intended it to be. And I truly believe that she is happy with the result. I also believe that should you choose to read Barbara's loving, despairing yet ultimately triumphant Odyssey, WHEN WAS IT I DARED TO DREAM, *The Journey of a Soul Incarnate*, you will not be disappointed.

John Flynn

Beloved Companion

It is 5:30 A.M. My clock radio has awakened me to the sounds of smooth jazz... and my body, heavy from sleep, heavy from Polio, moves, stretches and begins to nudge the covers away for more freedom. I know I will not rush this early morning rising ritual. Polio has taught me well to take all the time I need to notice each small detail of rising–my morning prayer and awareness of another day dawning. It will be a full thirty minutes before I am sitting in my wheelchair at exactly six o'clock. I have noticed each detail of moving from sleep to wakefulness, to reaching for my corset and handling that garment precisely, so that I will wear it comfortably until I remove it at the end of the day when I lie down again to sleep. My electric bed responds to the remote control in my hand and raises me to sitting when Susha, my cat friend of thirteen years, jumps up on the bed and tries to engage me in a snuggle. But, get out of my way Susha. You know I have to pay attention. I must transfer from this bed to my chair. I reach deliberately for the transfer board that I had carefully left in exactly the right spot the night before. I swing my left arm so that my hand rests on the back of the chair for support as I wriggle the rest of me closer to the edge of the bed. Susha rubs her body against my hip. I mischievously throw the covers over her and carefully place the board beneath my legs as I slide on to it toward the chair–inch by precalculated inches. Polio, my beloved companion, reminds me. "Pay attention. Take all the time you need to be safe" as I slide into–kind of fall into the seat of my chair and reach with my right hand for the edge of the board that gives me the solid stiffness I need to pull my body up straight. I catch my balance, position myself, pull the board away, unplug the charger that has recharged my batteries while I slept and reach for the detached arm rest that I secure in place before flipping the switch that gives my chair the signal to move. "You doin' okay?" Mary, readying herself for work, queries from the doorway–Mary Armato–my love, my dear friend, my neighbor, my traveling companion who often stays the night to offer assistance, if needed. "All set," I reply. It is now six o'clock a.m. as I roll away from the bedside toward the bathroom. I am prayerfully grateful that I am independent in all ADL "activities of daily living" i.e. toileting bathing, and dressing.

Today I am sixty. And today I share with you a love story. Today I will stop, notice, rejoice and say a morning prayer in praise of this constant one who is with me. This one who has held me as no other one has ever done. This one who placed me lovingly at the age of ten in the safety and security of the Iron Lung under the loving gazes, attention and care of expert Nurses and Doctors whose love and dutiful attention breathed life into the soul of a child. This one who gave me appropriate mentors and guides for a lifetime— caretakers and bosom friends with whom I learned to locomote and grow again in triumph.

Indeed, this is a love story.

PART ONE

Bulletproof

I am still whole. I am still connected to the rest of me. Here I am again–a new day. My arms, my legs and my body still joined together–strangely not moving, yet all there. I do not worry. They make all the decisions as they hover over me–discussing and deciding what to do with me. All I have to do is lie quiet and passive and watch as they deal with my body. I am the center of their attention as I pee, am bathed, comforted and arranged properly in this tank–this huge *Iron Lung* from which I hadn't been removed much since I got here–just opened up and looked at for a few minutes. I am breathing on my own during those few minutes. And now I am gently raised by people on either side of the tank and moved again through the opening. My head is separated from the rest of me and the mighty tank is rolled shut. The black pump at the other end roars IN AND OUT, IN AND OUT and the tank begins again to breathe for me. Ah, this pleases all of me very much. I am comfortable. And so I doze and sleep for a while. My day is full of surprises. And when I awake, hands are reaching in from the outside to exercise my arms and legs. To lift them and move them gently, passively, while someone else shows me cards that are arriving from neighbors and friends in Stoneham, Massachusetts. Surprises. Strange. All this attention. There is no rejection here. All I have to do is be passive–lie there with no movement. And these people gather around me and bring me cards, gifts and messages. People who never saw me before now notice me. A light now shines on me in this yellow tank. Day after day of surprises. I am lifted again from the safety of my tank to the rocking bed. I am small in the big bed. It rocks from head to toe. My head is rocked deep down and raised high up, down and up, down and up and I breathe in and out, in and out, as the bed rocks down and up, down and up. I look over at my tank from here–my big yellow tank. I am safe. I am passive. And I watch everyone busy around me. There are others here too in Division 36–Children and grownups. Like me, all of these people have polio too and no one knows why. No one knows where the polio comes from. Lots of people have polio. Some people die from it. And some people hardly ever know they had polio. Some, like me, get lots of polio. Most of the people here now don't have as much polio as I have. Yes, I have lots of polio.

Ma says it's because I went to the beach with Aunt Dot and got a chill. Dad thinks it's because the Dentist in Wakefield pulled my tooth out a few weeks before and it got infected. I think it is because I played naked in the woods with Timmy. I know that's really why. And that's really why no one tells. I don't tell. No one tells. And that's why no one tells how people get polio. People get polio by doing stuff with their bodies. Stuff you're told not to do. Fun stuff. Bad stuff. Like me and Timmy. It's weird because polio makes you a hero–a big star. Everyone notices you and sends you cards. And suddenly just because you have polio you are a big hero. The nuns ask you to pray for THEM, because they think the prayers of a sick child are the best. God listens to the prayers of a sick child. So the nuns are quick to ask for prayers, whereas before they never noticed me. I was nobody before I had polio. Now I'm a big hero. If they only knew. Those dumb nuns. I dislike them intensely. They are only interested in me now because I can pray for them–get them in good with God. They are really crazy. God knows and so do I. I try to hide from God these days because God knows how come I got polio. He knows, so I avoid Him. I don't go seeking Him out to pray. No way. I avoid all of that. And I especially hate the priest who comes from the mission church, who wants to hear my confession. I don't talk to him. He leans over my rocking bed and urges me to tell him my sins. He scares me to death. So I just stay passive and real quiet. If anyone around Division 36 really knew how I got polio I wouldn't be a hero anymore. Like those people with Leprosy– the people with polio would be cast away somewhere. Abandoned, like the Lepers. So it is best to be quiet. And eventually the priest will go away. And I won't pray for those awful nuns either.

The Iron Lung is my grand protector–makes me feel bulletproof. On its soft cushioned mattress, the big powerful machine holds me, engulfs me totally. Holds me completely as it breathes in and out–in and out in great swishes. Great powerful swishes. The huge black pump at the foot of the tank forces me to breathe–in and out–in and out. And all I have to do is lie there and the huge machine does it all. And no one says' "Go away." No one says, "Don't bother me." The People are all here coaxing me to eat– bathing me, turning me, moving my arms and my legs. I like them. So I let them. A brand new beginning. A new chance to start again. Glory! Glory! To start again. All over again. And I pretend not to remember, although to myself I do remember. I know.

They make comments–nice comments that I know aren't true. But to the new girl–not the old girl. I have to keep the old girl quiet–hidden, so they won't find her and reject her, like the others did...

Such great relief I felt when Polio claimed me for its own. An alien perhaps, but no longer rejected. Finally, fully embraced by something– the Iron Lung that accepted me from the git go without the vaguest hint of rejection. Didn't push me away like I was so used to, but opened its arms and folded me up inside its huge yellow self–safe inside this massive yellow solace that took over my breathing. Deep, deep, deep, deep down I am so relieved to be held–to be supported so–all the way through and through. So when "YOU" came into my room, to sit behind me, by the wall –"YOU" and Dad–"YOU" sit there still and cold, imprisoned and rejecting still–closed in–locked in with your worries and limitations. I'm in MY IRON LUNG. I no longer need "YOU." I have Polio now to embrace me totally. To be with me. My Iron Lung is stronger than "YOU" and will not reject me–will not turn me away. My Iron Lung will hold me and enfold me totally and it will even breathe for me. "YOU" can leave now. "YOU" can go home. I said to my nurse, "Tell them to go home." And I see "YOU" rise and leave,"YOU" and Dad– broken spirits–broken hearts–crushed. And I feel so sad for you." I ache inside for all you are not, as I settle into my soft cushioned Iron Lung. It breathes in and out, in and out. I am safe. I am saved. I am sheltered. I am protected. I am loved by my Iron Lung. I am possessed by Polio– embraced totally, all of me, head to toe–finally contained within myself to a place "YOU" will never come–never be. Not "YOU" Not "YOU" ever.

Like I said... *Bulletproof.*

Moving

Moving out was the hardest thing I had ever done in my life. It was Holy Week. Ma was eighty-six years old. Her short term memory was gone and I had to go. Ma and I had lived together for all of my fifty-two years. Maybe it was because I had Polio when I was ten and Ma thought she had to take care of me until I moved out, so she could go ahead and die. Maybe I stayed so long because Ma was the adult child of an alcoholic mother, which made me the adult child of a tee totaling Irish Catholic martyr and I wanted to make the last of her life better than the first had been. I don't know. I just know that it was Holy Thursday and my pal Ethel had got out of teaching school at noontime and came over with her daughter Jannique (my Godchild) and they both walked right on in past Ma and past my brother Paul–a Maryknoll Priest, who was sitting in the mauve swivel rocker with his prayer book on his lap and his back to all the action. Ethel and Jannique went into my bedroom and removed clothes from my closet and carried them out to the car. They made trip after trip until they couldn't get any more in.

On Friday, Good Friday, Ken and Bill came by and took my stereo equipment and entertainment center out, leaving Ma's TV on a smaller table. Ma kept up her pleasant smile for the company. She hardly knew what was happening. I knew what was happening. For days I had cried and cried and cried to and for myself. I couldn't believe I was actually moving out of my Mother's house–out of the home we had shared at 150 North Street in Stoneham Mass. and had taken care of for so long.

On Saturday, *Holy Saturday*, while Ma was getting her hair done, more help arrived to take out the sofa, my computer, printer and writing table. They reassembled it all in the new apartment which was only one and a half miles away in the south end of town. My friend Marie had asked me not to ask her to take stuff out of the house in front of Ma. She said she would make pillows and chair sets with some material that a friend had picked out.

It was April and Ma's health had been failing for a long time. The aneurism in her abdomen pressed on her sciatic nerve causing chronic pain. My sister Peggy and I had asked Paul to come home from his Missionary work to help out. Earlier in his spiritual journey he had been a Seminarian with the Mill Hill Fathers, then on to St. Louis University and later in London, England for three years of *Major Seminary* training. Then for seventeen years he made his home among the people in Taiwan whose language he learned to speak fluently.

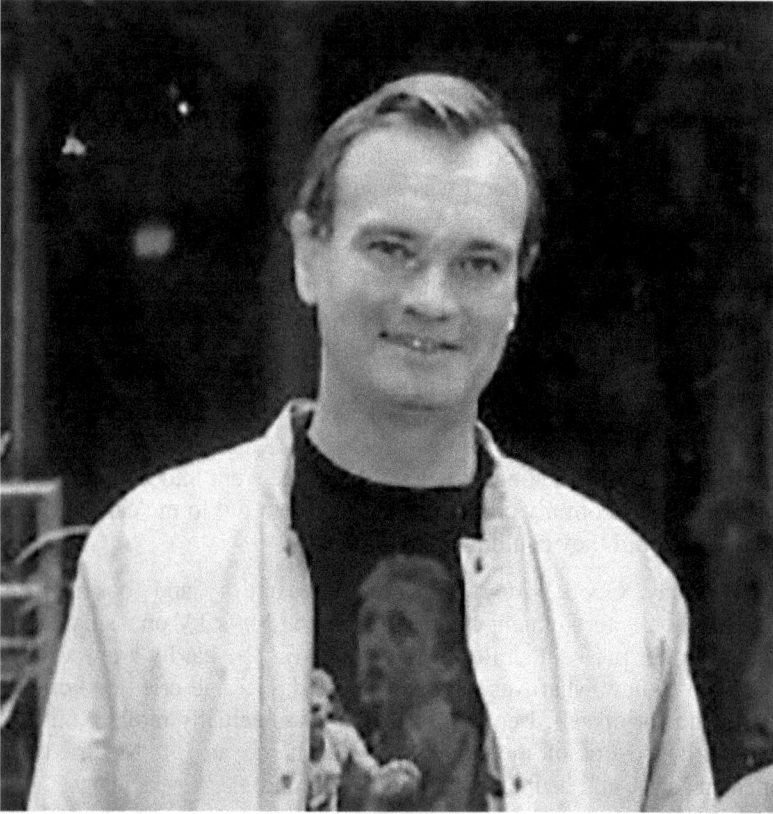

Father Paul Duffy

Paul was a great help. He took care of Ma during the day while I went to work at Mass Rehab and Peg helped out with the meals and some cleaning. The three of us working together provided 24 hours of positive care and attention and for a while Ma's health did stabilize. But Paul was scheduled to leave May 5th for a Forty Day Retreat in Canada.

Back in January, one of Peggy's grown daughters, Sharon, had called me from her home in Kansas.

"What are you going to do when Gram dies?" Are you going to move out?

"Gram's Will is clear about that," I replied. "She and Grampy wrote the Will twenty-five years ago and Gram reviewed it three years ago. The house is left to the three of us, but I have a *Life Estate* which allows me to live in the house here in Stoneham for as long as I need to, or want to."

Ma and I had continued to live in the house after Dad died in 1975. They had purchased the home in 1963 because it was wheelchair accessible and I had graduated from college and needed to learn how to drive and get a job. That was before the days of Independent Living for people with disabilities and before the days of Supplemental Security Income or Social Security Disability Insurance. Ma was very supportive in all of this and with the assistance of a local Realtor they found the three bedroom ranch just one mile away from the old house at 37 Cottage Street that Ma and Dad had built when they got married in 1935, following the Depression.

Dad had retired and drove me to work every day and also drove me to Northeastern University for my Graduate School classes at night in Burlington until I got my Driver's License in 1967 and got my own car. After Dad died Ma and I wanted to stay living in the house and with our combined income we knew we could handle it. The year after Dad died we added a sundeck. And a couple of years after that we had the kitchen remodeled so I could be a fully functional homemaker, as Ma's health began to show signs of aging. We spoke every now and then about other options and each time we re-decided that it was her desire and mine to stay living in the house. I had my work and life and she was very active as well. She went to the Sixty-Plus Club and every Friday and met with her friends at the Redstone shopping center for lunch. I felt truly independent. Ma did her thing and I did mine. I taught and did counseling work, traveled and enjoyed my friends. At that time Peggy, her husband Paul and their three young children–Sharon, Susan and John had moved from Atlanta back to Stoneham which enabled the kids to grow up right around the corner from us. Unfortunately, Peggy held on to lifelong resentments through those years and beyond. She divorced her husband, Paul Murphy and did not remarry. She worked hard but did not like her job much. She said I was the lucky one because I had an education and a career. So like I mentioned, when my youngest niece, Sharon, (then married) called me on the phone from Kansas I wasn't really too surprised by her question, "What are you going to do when Gram dies?" Although, it still raised all my fears again and even though I told her that I was going to continue doing the same things I had been doing, she pressed on, "But Mama is going to get her share of the house when Gram dies," isn't she," she insisted.

"It doesn't quite work that way," I told her and I explained again about Ma's Will and the Life Estate.

"But Mama says she's going to get her share of the house and I want to know what you are going to do." Because she was acutely sensitive to the interpersonal dynamics of our family and knew just what buttons to push to make my head spin and my blood pressure rise, I was worried about the conversation, so an hour later I called her sister, Susan, who usually distanced herself from controversy and thought things out calmly.

"Please don't be mad at Sharon," she said. "She's trying to prepare you. We both are. We love you and we care about you and we're worried about you. Mama is talking about getting her share of the house when Gram dies and she expects Paul will agree with her. And we want you to take care of yourself."

When Peggy's son, John, came in to visit later on that same day I needed to hear his spin on this and sure enough he had been hearing the same thing.

"Listen, not to worry," he said. Mama... Peggy... will always be Peggy."

But worry I did! So I asked Paul, "What is the story? What have you been hearing ?"

"Listen," he said. "I'm home to take care of Ma and afterwards I'm on a plane back to Taiwan. Meanwhile I can put up with all the B.S. because I know it's only temporary."

End of conversation. Sharon and Susan were right. I needed to *take care of myself.*

Peggy would come over to look after Ma–give her a bath and bring her to Holy Communion. Then she would come back to get Paul for 5:30 Mass. "Are you ready, Hon?" she would call out to Paul as she entered the kitchen. If I happened to be on the phone, she would yell out, "Where's my brother! I want to talk to my brother!" I became invisible. Paul saw to it that he wasn't at home as much as possible. And Peggy let me know that she came in and out only to take care of Ma. I felt more and more estranged–a stranger in my own home. Susan and Sharon were older then and busy with their families. They pulled back and didn't call or come by much after that.

But when they had said, "Take care of yourself." essentially they meant it as a warning–*Mama will win. Get out.* They had made it quite clear that they were in agreement. But how could I get out? Where would I go? None of my friend's houses were accessible. "Get an apartment," someone said. My mind fought back. How on earth can I do that? Why should I do that? This is my home! Accessible apartments have long waiting lists. I've never lived alone–never been on my own. Fear rushed in on me like a Tsunami. I needed help. I needed to protect myself. Ma was becoming more and more childlike–repeating, "My three wonderful children. What would I do without my three wonderful children." I felt like I was living in the "Glass Menagerie." I HAD TO GET OUT! Such a great urgency to go and there was no place *to* go. And Paul was leaving for Canada. Actually Paul left when he was eighteen and never really looked back. His physical presence since then had simply been that–a physical presence.

Finally, I hired a Family Counselor, Stephen Maurer, to listen and guide me through this time of crisis.

He said, "There is a Chinese character for the idea of crisis and it contains two elements. One is for danger–the other for opportunity. In every crisis there is both danger and opportunity."

I went to a Lawyer who explained more extensively to me the meaning of the *Life Estate*, which gives a disabled person the right to continue living in a mutually owned home, despite the needs of other siblings.

I turned to Ethel and her husband Phil Holland.

"Don't worry," they said, "You can come and live with us." And although the offer was kind and comforting, the vision of their tiny three room apartment, them, me and my electric wheelchair didn't exactly open up a spacious field of hope. Finally I called the Independent Living Center and asked about apartments and I got the name of a Realtor specializing in accessible housing.

I submitted my application on a Monday and by Thursday morning Mary Jewett called me and said, "I have just what you're looking for right here in Stoneham–a wonderful wheelchair accessible garden apartment in your price range and available now. Do you want to come over and look at it?" "YES, today," I said. It began to happen almost immediately. But how could this be? Clients wait for years to get what they need. Accessible apartments aren't that readily available. This is eerie. And just a few miles away from this house. Remembering Stephen's piece of wisdom that in every crisis there is both danger and opportunity, I had to see this incredible possibility. I saw it that very day and the apartment was wonderful. It was on the ground floor with two exterior entrances, a parking space, a fully accessible kitchen and bathroom. Could it be? That opportunity??? I thought, "No, this is crazy. Why am I doing this?" I went home for supper and Paul was there.

"I looked at an apartment today," I said. "Why?" he asked. "You don't have to move out. Don't worry. Peggy will let you live here. Give her a chance to be kind to you. She doesn't want the house. She has a house. She just wants as much control over it as you have. If she wants the house let her have it. She'll let you live in it."

My mind raced. Yes, I loved my dear brother. But just listen to that–anything for peace, just to keep the peace. Let Peggy be the matriarch.

She can take over where Ma left off. Let her take care of you. My protection antennae shot up. I knew I needed to protect myself, so I went back to Stephen again and with his kindness and gentle wisdom he told me to move toward the Light. He saw excitement in my response to the apartment. The more we talked about it, the more real it became. And when I left him I knew that I was going to move out. I was going to move out of my mother's house! How could this be? Ma was so frail.

And Stephen said "You are giving your mother a great gift. You are showing her that you can make it on your own without her. You are making it possible for her to finally let go of that tedious, all-consuming job. She has taken care of you since your birth and so much more so since the onset of the Polio. You have been her sick child and she has not let go of life because she doesn't think you can take care of yourself. Moving out into your own apartment will show her that you can take care of yourself and she will be able to let go. Don't you see? Everyone will benefit. Peggy can take care of her as much as she wants and a plan for your Mother's care will allow Paul to go on his Retreat and then back to Taiwan."

Through the man's thoughtful words, the truth of the matter emerged and became as clear as sunlight. Ma and I had given all we had to give to each other. It was time to move on.

Suddenly everything within and without became possible. I felt an overwhelming sense of freedom and excitement. There was a solution where there was none before! My friends agreed and said they would help. What would Ma say? And Peggy? Paul? Susan, John and Sharon? What would they say about this, now that it was a definite possibility. Ma regained her old strength for awhile and said, "Over my dead body you'll move out! This is your home! I'll not hear of it!!" I said nothing to Peggy and asked Paul to carry the news to her. Stephen suggested a meeting with the three of us and Peggy and Paul agreed. We needed a plan for Ma's care while Paul went on Retreat. Stephen made some observations, "Good fences make good neighbors," he said, "Distance will be good for all of you."

Ethel and Phil came over to disassemble my bed and take the rest of my bedroom furniture to the new place. I would sleep there for the first time that Saturday night. During the week, Ma and I drove to our favorite spot by Lake

Quannapowitt in Wakefield, where over the years she and I had spent many hours together and that was where we finally had a total and serious talk about my new apartment.

"I don't know why, Ma, I really don't know why... at this time in our lives... if you were me Ma, what would you do?"

"If I had your courage, I'd do the same thing," she said. "And you don't have to know why. No one else knows why either. Peggy and Paul had their chance to get on with their lives. You deserve that chance too."

I couldn't believe what I was hearing. Was Ma really supporting me in this most incredible move! Indeed. She certainly was. She loved me with all she had, and I loved her with all I had. There was so much of the unknown that lay ahead. There was excitement and bouts of unrelenting anxiety.

That Holy Saturday night Ma said it was her curiosity that brought her to my apartment. I made her a cup of tea. She walked through the rooms. "I'd like to turn down your bed. Do you mind?" she asked.

"Go ahead Ma. It's okay. Go ahead."

It was her final gesture. On Easter Sunday morning I awoke with joy in a place of my own. I was safe. Over and over and over, I repeated the words, "I am safe. I am safe." Three weeks later on Mother's Day, Ma died of a stroke, having been hospitalized for five days. She was eighty six. It was Springtime.

One year later in time for Easter Sunday, I returned home for good. The house had again been renovated to keep in sync with my ability to function independently with even more ease and comfort than before. I was safe. I was loved. I shared life with my friends. Paul called frequently and visited often for dinner when he was on leave from his missionary work. Although I had little contact with Peggy and her children during that coming home period, I was grateful for the past and mindful in the present. I had finally realized that with God, friends and a few neatly placed purveyors of wisdom like Stephen Maurer, all things are possible. But it also takes my will and my willingness to participate in full.

I am alive today
a continuation of the women before me
Ma before me and Nana before her
Peggy Ann and cousin Bette Jean
Women before me
And I before Susan and Sharon
And they before Cara, Kailey and Kristen,
Courtney, Sara and Kimberly
A steady stream of women
I exist in this chain of life-giving
Women To be life
To give life
I breathe in and I breathe out
I hold my life in my arms
I give thanks and praise to the Goddess
Within.

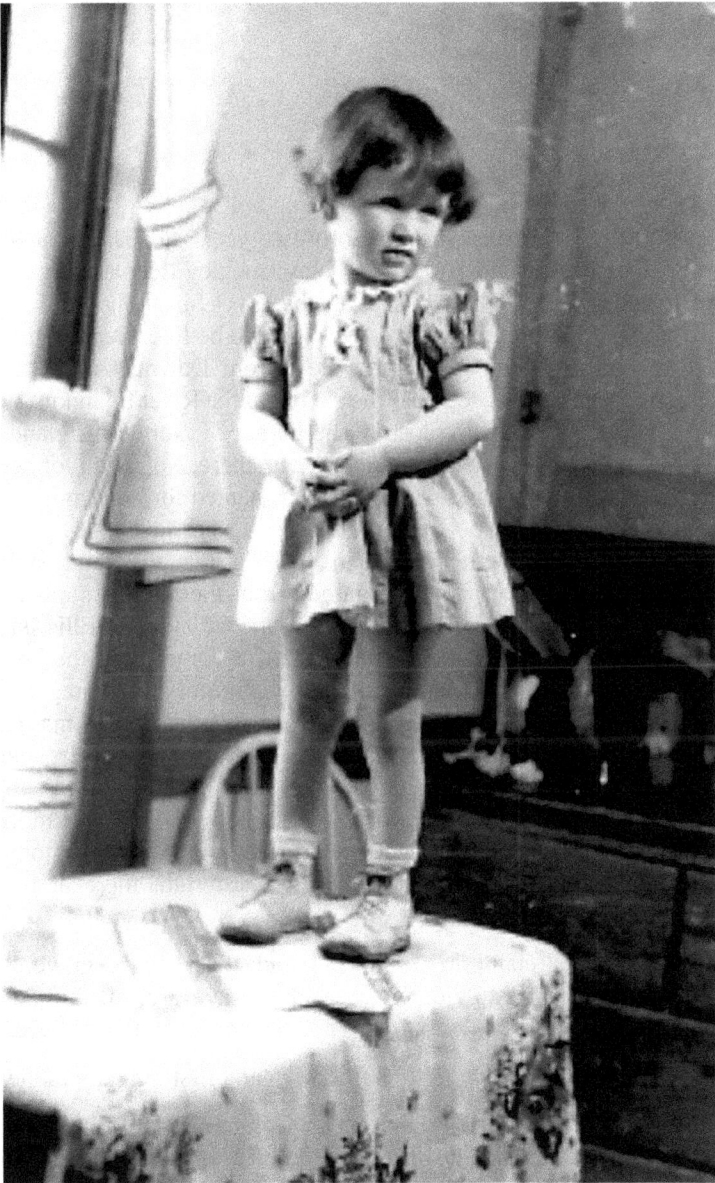

Barbara on the table, aged 4.

Beginnings

Nana gave birth to Ma when she was forty-two years old. The same age Ma was when she gave birth to Paul. Ann Foley Buckley Lee would get lost in her reverie and tell how she stepped over the River Shannon and was proud of it. She was proud of much of her life struggle to be free. Her struggle to be independent and not a burden. Ann Foley, from Dawra, County Cavern, Ireland, born years ago in 1863 near the source of the River Shannon. Way up in the hills of County Cavern close to the border of Northern Ireland. Poor then, they were sheep herders. Not much else up there. Not much for her large family of brothers and sisters. Ann the Tailor, named for her family's trade. Bright, poetic and romantic–good at memorizing her texts. At age sixteen when she heard her brothers moan their fate of growing old and paying off their sisters' dowries, Ann stole the money from the kitchen cupboard and booked passage for America. At sixteen she arrived alone at Ellis Island to find her relatives in New York and to work as a domestic in the homes of New York's well established families. Ann was bright and courageous. She took risks and she married Dan Buckley. He was a handsome maître-de at a fine New York restaurant. She managed to return alone to Ireland, still nursing her first baby, to visit her mother. Still young, she ran through the Irish hillside burying her bare toes into her beloved sod once more. Her mother called her back to their cottage to nurse her infant–a moment of bliss, only to be followed by the infant's death right there at home in Ireland.

On a visit to Ireland in 1990, I found that baby's grave. "Most assuredly" the local priest said, "Here in this graveyard, all the Catholics were buried here then. 1885 or so, you say? Aye, most assuredly here."

The grave of my grandmother's first born and first of many to die.

Ann Foley Buckley left Ireland, never to return again. She came back to New York to a faithless husband and the birth of more babies. Alice in 1890. Mildred was born two years after Alice. All of Nana's other babies born of her marriage to Dan, died. Some of pneumonia, some of syphilis and others were still born. Dan died when Mildred was three and Alice was five. The three of them, Ann with her tiny daughters, Alice and Mildred, moved from New York to Lynn, Massachusetts to begin again and Mildred died, too. "All you have now is me," Alice told Ma. And they created a bond that lasted a lifetime–linked by humor, poetry and courage–courage to go on. Patrick J. Lee helped with that. Pat, the Butcher–a Kerryman born in Dingle, County Kerry in 1860. Another marriage and more babies. Ma (Dorothy Margaret) was born in 1905 on June 24th when Alice was fifteen. A son Stephen Martin was born on the Feast of St. Stephen, December 26 and died before his first birthday.

Women Survivors

Fierce Broken Alienated,

Even from themselves

Most deeply

from themselves

Generations of women Lost

In the hills of County Cavern Ireland

The burial of a baby in 1885

Surely the deepening of grief

The path to despair

All the while

Holding on to a Faith in a God

And in a Church that reinforces

Suffering and death as the way To Eternal Salvation

God loves those who suffer most

God gives the hardest burdens

To those he loves the most,

So all that pain–all that suffering

Is swallowed like the Communion wafer

To sustain life

Little bits and pieces of life.

At Christmas, Easter, the 4th of July and Thanksgiving, Ann Foley Buckley Lee found relief in Whiskey. It numbed her broken heart with days and nights of total numbness. Followed by guilt, sorrow and more promises. brought to an end only by senile dementia in her eighties...

Her true obituary would read:

Ann Foley Buckley Lee

was a member

of the lay religious order of St. Francis...

The Third Order of St. Francis

Abstinence from

meat Fasting and Abstaining

Prayer and Penance

A lifelong numbness

To bury alive

The pain

of too many dead babies

... and so Ma grew up encompassed by pain and unpredictability, bereft of a normal mother's expression of love and kindness–a broken mother who held too much grief already to risk any more.

16 Perley Street

Every Sunday afternoon at three o'clock, we drove in Dad's 1934 black Ford to West Lynn to visit Nana, Grampa, Aunt Alice and Uncle Mike at 16 Perley Street that Ma referred to with pride as "Lee's Block." Ma and her family lived there in the three decker, where she had been born and where she lived until she married Dad in 1935. We stopped on the way to buy harlequin ice cream–in brick form.

The ride to West Lynn was always the same route. Dad loved to drive. He had a great sense of direction and we rarely got lost. In all of the forty years Dad drove, he never had an accident. The Ford always looked brand new because Dad took pride in his car. He cleaned it regularly with a soft chamois cloth and kept it simonized. He kept the engine in good condition by figuring out ahead what was likely to go wrong and had many of the parts replaced before they broke down. No one ever drove Dad's car but him. Ma never renewed her license after she was married and gave up her job as a Stenographer.

Dad said she didn't need to drive–that he'd take her where she needed to go. Dad's car was Dad's car! It was their pattern. Dad held to what was his and Ma held to what was hers.

After Sunday Mass we would have Sunday dinner at one o'clock and after Ma cleaned up the kitchen, we were on our way. Dad drove through Wakefield Square down Water Street into Saugus, past a rickety old house where an old fella sold popcorn. Peggy and I sang a made up song about the popcorn man. "Popcorn man, popcorn man. Won't you be my popcorn man." On Walnut Street we drove past the Reservoir and the Lynn Woods, took a right on to Myrtle Street and a left at Howard's Market and finally a right on to 16 Perley Street.

Ma took pride in the gray three story building–the way she took pride in Nana's courage to invest in Lee's block, even though she knew Nana was counting on her to help pay the mortgage for the whole thing. That was why Nana discouraged Ma from going on to high school after the eighth grade. Instead, Ma went to Burdett Business School to get the education that would lead her to a job that would better help pay the mortgage. So when Ma was seventeen she got her first job as a stenographer in Boston. Most of her friends who had quit school in the eighth grade, went to work at the GE plant. Ma felt special and privileged to be a secretary working in Boston, even though she was scared about it at first. And Ma so much shared Nana's pride in owning Lee's Block, she went on to support the block until she married Dad, two days before she turned thirty.

Dad parked in the long, narrow driveway to the left of the three decker. A single car garage was at the very end and a narrow cement walkway ran between the driveway and the tall gray wooden house. There was enough room for Aunt Alice's pink and white Peonies. There were porches on the front and porches on the back of the house on all three floors. We trudged up the inside back stairway to the second floor and always inhaled the same musty, cold, damp smell that led us up the stairs and finally into the back hall that led into the kitchen. Everything about the old house was wooden–wooden in a different way from our house on Cottage Street in Stoneham. This wood was old like Nana and Grampa and they smelled just like the old house.

A door led from the back hallway on to the back porch. All the doors were dark brown wood and the back hall was cool in the summer and cold in the winter. Out on the porch the clothes line was strung over to the garage on a pulley. Dad would say, "Watch out! Be careful!" because he didn't trust the old wooden railings to stay put if we leaned too hard against them. The brown wooden door to the kitchen was shut when we arrived. We knocked before entering the large kitchen.

Nana sat in her big dark brown wicker chair by the window wearing a flowered apron that covered her house dress and stopped at the top of her knees. Her knees ached from arthritis and she would rub them to ease the pain. We had to be careful not to touch her because when we did, she would wince with pain, causing us to pull quickly back. Nana's body was of the mesomorph variety–square and wide and she fit snug in her chair with her white hair piled on top of her head.

Grampa sat on the couch against the wall under the wind up clock with Nancy, his tiny smooth haired fox terrier beside him. He sat there Sunday after Sunday keeping watch on Nana and also kept his eye on Aunt Alice and Uncle Mike. Grampa was tall and thin, with gray-white hair neatly combed back and a gray mustache. He wore wire frame glasses and always wore his good pants and vest on Sundays. The vest had pockets for his round, gold watch and tobacco pouch. The watch fit comfortably

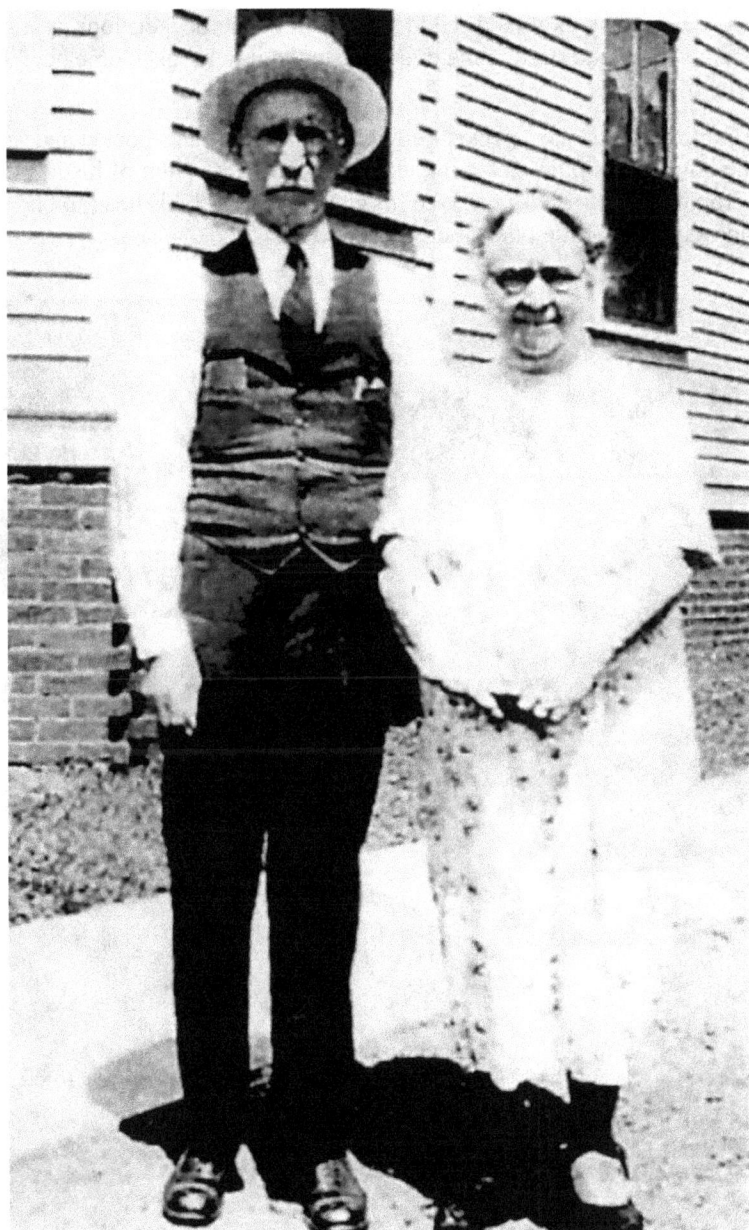

Grandpa and Nana

into the palm of his big hand. He'd slip it out of the pocket, look at it, then look at me, wink and beckon me over to listen to it ticking. "Come here, little one," he'd say.

Grampa would take a pocket knife out of his back pants pocket and scrape out the bowl of his pipe, knocking its contents into the palm of his left hand, then drop it into the ash tray next to his chair. He'd cock his head to one side, nod and say "Aye, little one, sit down over here."

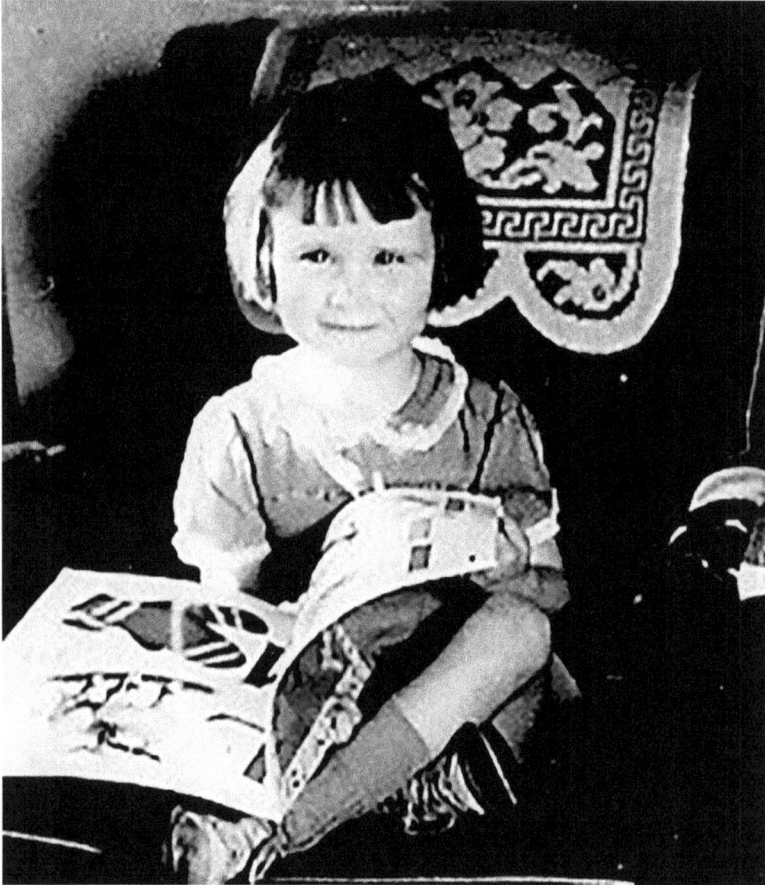

Barbara age 3

And he'd tell me a story. I liked Grampa. I liked that he was tall and had nice eyes. His eyes told me how very much he liked me. They sparkled.

While Grampa talked to me, Nancy would twitch all over as she looked out the window and caught a glimpse of another dog yipping and yapping and trotting along the sidewalk. Grampa would say "sic 'em, Boy, sic 'em!" even though Nancy was a girl.

Aunt Alice would make conversation with Ma and Peggy would quickly disappear. Uncle Mike stayed in the dining room sitting in one of the large over-stuffed chairs by the bay windows where the afternoon sun streamed in to warm the old place. The Sunday paper lay on his lap and on the floor beside the chair. He would slump down and seem to be asleep. I didn't like Uncle Mike. I remember Ma saying she didn't like "Mike" either. Alice and Mike. That's how Ma referred to them. They married later in life–eloped before Ma and Dad got married. They both worked at GE in the factory section and they had no children. Mike was English and being a Kerryman, Grampa didn't like him much and Nana didn't trust him either. Their Irish roots were dug too deep to allow much room for trusting an Englishman. Ma said that Aunt Alice only married him because she didn't get any other offers.

The visits to Perley Street on Sundays were joyful for me until one afternoon when Uncle Mike called me over to sit on his lap and I felt his fingers groping between my legs. An icy-like terror raced through me, making me feel that I was bad. I ran away from him and moved toward the others for comfort without saying anything. Ma said "Go on now and play. I'm busy." Peggy said "Get away you little pig." Dad said "Come over here *Stevie*. (Dad's nickname for me) He put a gentle arm around my shoulder, giving me the shelter I needed at that moment. He was so clean–so pure. I felt ashamed. I crawled close to him and slunk down deep inside myself and stayed that way for a long time.

On most of our Sunday visits Dad would go in the dining room to sit with Uncle Mike and read the paper, too. The living room was dark and uninviting and we only went in there on holidays. Mostly we stayed in the kitchen and dining room. Eventually the ice cream would be cut in slices and we'd eat it with plain Vanilla cookies. Nana had shiny new pennies for us and she counted them out, "One for you and one for you and another one for you and another one for you..." Grampa watched and teased and tried to take away our attention. Nana would say "Stop teasing." Grampa's teasing was fun. I didn't want him to stop. Grampa was the only really good thing for me about that Sunday ritual. He would cock his head to one side, wink and say "Aye, little one, Aye."

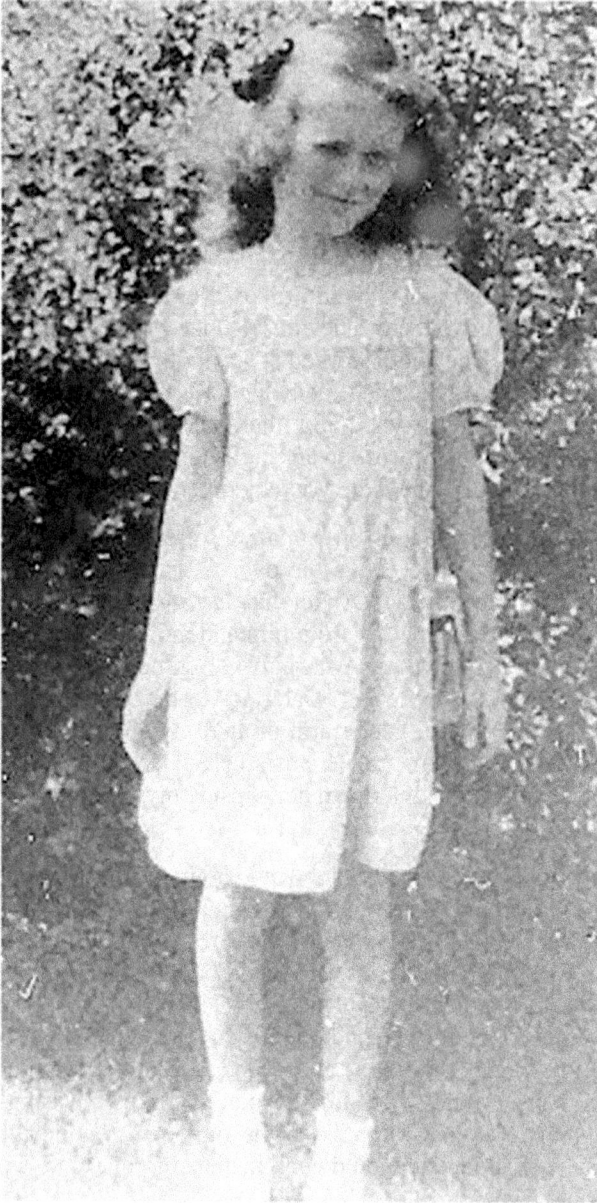

Peggy

Peggy hated those Sundays. And she hated Uncle Mike too, but never said why. The visits didn't stop until after Nana and Grampa died. Nana died two days after Christmas in 1947. I was eight years old and in the third grade. Peggy was eleven, Paul was almost one. Nana was eighty-three. She was waked in the living room at 16 Perley Street and we had to turn off the Christmas Lights. Nana was laid out in the brown robes of the Third Order of Saint Francis. Her casket was in front of the bay windows but the room was mostly dark. Ma and Aunt Alice took turns staying up all night so Nana wouldn't be left alone. Dad took me and Peggy home and because Peggy was almost twelve, she was in charge of me and Paul while Ma buried Nana. She was buried on the First Friday of January. Grampa was buried four months later on the First Friday in May. It had been their religious practice to keep holy the First Fridays in remembrance of the Crucifixion which had happened on a Friday... They kept The Faith.

I felt sad when Grampa died. I sat at the kitchen table the morning of his Wake and said I didn't want to go. Ma objected until Dad said I didn't have to go and Ma finally gave in and said I didn't have to go. I was glad Dad stuck up for me. I just felt too sad to go. I remembered Nana in the casket in the living room in front of the bay window and I didn't want to see Grampa there. I wanted to see him sitting on the couch in the kitchen, calling me over, cocking his head to one side with a wink saying, "Aye, little one, Aye." On Memorial Day, a few weeks later, Ma cried as we walked away from his grave. She was holding my hand, "Don't tell your father," she said.

Siobhan

"Mark my words, Siobhan, you'll not get your share." Grampa called Ma Siobhan (pronounced *shiv* + *awn*) the Irish form of Joan, meaning "God is gracious." Ma quoted him years later: "Mark my words, Siobhan, you'll not get your share!" Grampa was talking about the three decker. Nana wanted them to live there all together–Nana, Grampa, Alice and Mike and Ma and Dad. But Ma and Dad would have none of it. They were satisfied having a place of their own where they were their own boss and were not at the beck and call of Alice and Mike. So, they said no. Aunt Alice and Uncle Mike made their home with Nana and Grampa and years later when Nana was very old, had a stroke and needed care, Aunt Alice quit her job at the GE plant and stayed home to take care of her mother.

Alice and Mike wanted Nana and Grampa to turn the house over to them, because if the house were not in Nana and Grampa's name, she and Mike would be entitled to health care benefits. So the discussion came about and Nana said, "As long as Dorothy gets her share." And Alice said, "It wouldn't be Christian not to give Dorothy her share." And Grampa said, "Mark my words, Siobhan, you'll not get your share." And Ma said, "Of course I will Grampa." But the house was put in Alice and Mike's name.

After Nana and Grampa died, Mike sold the house to his niece, Kathleen, along with most of what was in the house. Ma found out about it after the fact, when Alice told her that she and Mike were moving into the housing for the Elderly. Aunt Alice claimed to be Grampa's only heir–his only next of kin. In fact she was his step daughter and Ma was his only actual next of kin. Ma got left out, except for a life insurance policy that named her as beneficiary. That summer Alice and Mike went to Europe for three months.

At home there was a great deal of talk about Ma not getting her share and Alice did her best to avoid Ma. When Ma did go to visit her, Alice trembled and shook all over and Ma was afraid she'd have a nervous breakdown. As it was, Alice wound up in the hospital for nerves and Ma decided to let the whole thing go and not to fight for the share she knew was hers. She said she felt bad for Alice, because she had been through some awful rough times with Nana's drinking. Ma remembered Alice's younger days and her fits of hysteria. And besides the trouble with her nerves, she was considerably less than pretty and didn't have many boyfriends, or girfriends. Ma remembered Nana's bouts with the bottle and said, "Alice got the worst of that."

There were other reasons for Ma's ultimate generosity toward Alice. When Ma was a small child, it was Alice who provided gentleness and generosity toward her. It was Alice who brought her books to read and took her to the Library. She tried to make up for Ma's barren, disappointing Christmases with toys, dolls and books. Alice had gone to work in the shoe factory when she was fourteen, a year before Ma was born. It was later that she worked at the GE plant and did that for many years until she quit to take care of Nana. Nana was senile in those last few years of her life and most of the time didn't know who Alice was, or Ma, or any of us. When Nana became senile, Alice was finally able to keep the bottle away from her. Senility took its place in the final numbing process.

Through the years Ma had witnessed the special relationship Alice had with Nana. How they shared jokes, enjoying a common sense of humor. They also shared a love of poetry and Irish music. We all respected Ma for not demanding her share. Ma shone. The fact that she didn't fight for her rightful share demonstrated a prime virtue in her character. It was the right thing to do. It was the noble thing to do. "After all," she said, "I have my own home and family and poor Alice never had it easy. All she has left is Mike and he's not worth having anyways."

After Nana and Grampa had passed and the house was sold, Ma and Aunt Alice drifted apart. It was 1949. I was ten. And when Ma got the money from Grampa's Insurance, Dad bought the only new car he ever owned–a gray two door Plymouth coupe. And in August that summer we went to Island Falls, Maine, for Dad's two week vacation. Later, many years later, after Mike died, Ma and Alice renewed their old relationship and became friends once again. In 1973 Aunt Alice died and left all her money to Ma. That was when Ma finally got *her* share.

The Babies

"My baby buntin'
Daddy's gone a'huntin'
To catch a little rabbit skin
To wrap my baby buntin' in"

Ma sang and rocked me in her lap as Peggy curled under her blankets. Other times when Dad worked overtime, Ma read Uncle Wiggly stories at bed time.

"Keep her in the sun until she turns red," the doctors told Ma in the Spring of 1940. So Ma did as the doctors ordered and she sat in the sun wearing her house dress covered with an apron, as she held me clothed only in a diaper. The sunshine did it Ma said. I believe the holding nourished me in 1940 when I would stop eating, which ma said was often. Ma said I would close my lips and hold them shut tight against feeding.

Doctor's Orders forced Ma to stop cleaning the house and hold her baby. Maybe the sunshine soaked its way into Ma's soul too. We got along like that–forced into needing (to feed) each other–symbiotically benefitting beyond our mutual resistance. Doctor's Orders crashed into Ma's tightly scheduled routine. "You must pay attention," doctors demanded.

Peggy was three years and three months old when I was born in August 1939. She hated me from the start. Long before I was born, Peggy screamed at Ma in angry outbursts! She crashed into Ma's daydreams with misbehavior–insisting–demanding Ma's attention. She scratched the face of one tiny visitor. She pulled the ribbons out of a neighbor child's hair. "Pay attention to me!," her behavior screamed. Ma paid attention by screaming back at her–threatening her–making her come into the house. Punishing her. But Peggy continued–yea increased the bad behavior more and more. She would race around the dining room table to escape Ma's wrath. Ma's screaming words flew across the room at her. "STOP! I SAID! STOP!" Ma would wave the hair brush above her head ready to hurl it at her. They grew

30

to hate each other. Peggy's face would freeze in an expression of deep and painful hurt. When I was born, Peggy couldn't abide all the attention I was getting, so she turned her rage toward me as well as Ma. I was scared to death of both of them. I stopped eating at six months and again at eight months. *Feeding problems*, the hospital Discharge Summary said in February of 1940. And again in April. While at Children's Hospital there were no feeding problems and I gained weight. So there was no reason, medically, or physically, why as an infant I did not eat. The story Ma told was that Peggy had a cold. The baby caught her cold and developed pneumonia. No one had bothered to read what the discharge summary said. And when Ma would hold me in the sunlight, Peggy looked on with seething, snarling, growling anger growing inside.

The Seasons

Spring on Cottage Street

I loved spring almost more than anything and I loved the brave purple violets that grew out of the cracks in the concrete that anchored the stones in the wall bordering the sidewalk. As soon as spring sprung I would walk up and down Cottage Street by myself, when the moist earth had a certain smell to it and there was dampness all around. I walked along the concrete sidewalk careful not to step on the cracks and bring bad luck. And there they were–the purple violets bursting through the cracks in the concrete–their rich green leaves pushing them up and out! Yes, there they were once again–peeking through the stone wall, thriving in that most unlikely place. I stopped, looked and noticed, touching them gently, but leaving them unmolested where they grew. Brave and strong, they struggled to life through the cracks. I needed to see how the violets grew, so I too could grow through the cracks in the concrete, like they did.

Winter on Cottage Street

I was seven and several weeks before Christmas, I was with Ma at a house on Main Street that in the 1940s specialized in Children's furniture and wooden toys. A small wooden rocking chair in the window captured my undivided, loving attention. The house was an important historical site in Stoneham. It had a sign on the outside describing its role in the Civil War as part of the underground railway for black slaves escaping to freedom in Canada. There was an underground passage beneath the house and the run-away slaves found safety and lodging there on their perilous journey. I stood beside Ma dreamily gazing at the rocking chair and the wooden doll's cradle beside it. On Christmas morning under the tree I found that same rocking chair and also the cradle with a baby doll in it. Ma told me Santa Claus had brought them.

Ma would be lost in her reverie when she wasn't cleaning and shining everything. An invisible wall surrounded her, kept her out of reach. I was four and remember one cold day I was feeling lonely, wanting to be close to her. "Go outside and play," she said, "Don't bother me now. Go out!" So I did. I stepped out on the back steps into the snow without my winter coat and heard the door click shut behind me. Peggy and all the other kids were in school. I stood on the top step shivering and heard Christmas songs coming from the radio through the closed door. It was getting real cold, but I wasn't strong enough to turn the doorknob and let myself in. Ma didn't hear me call out for her and I thought how nice and warm it would be if I was upstairs in the bedroom while she was dry mopping and dusting, or while she was sitting on the side of the bed looking at her stuff. I started to cry, but stopped right away when I heard Gene Autry singing, "You better watch out, you better not pout...you better not cry, I'm tellin' you why–Santa Claus is coming to town." It was cold inside and cold outside. I was cold, but the cold was not much compared to being lonely that day. Finally, Peggy came home from school, kicked open the door and went inside. She stood by the open door. "Hurry up you little pig," she said. "You want to freeze the whole house?"

When I was eight I went sledding down Rotundi's hill flopped down on my belly on my Flexible Flier with a kid on my back. WHIZZZZZ! Down the hill, over the bumps we went. The long sled took the two of us with ease 'til we came to a natural stop at the bottom of the hill. We picked up the sled and trudged back up the hill. I wore black buckled-up galoshes, navy blue leggings and a matching wool parka. We got to the top of the hill and turned...I started to run with the sled in my hands, ready to crash down onto the snow covered ground...plop...I landed belly down on my sled and my friend jumped... plop... belly down on top of me... WAAAMP! Good thing he's littler than me. We flew down over the bumps–faster and faster and faster, until suddenly we hit a dry spot of–GRASS and WHAMMM! My face smacked into the metal front part of the sled and my friend toppled over into a snow pile. Bleeding from the mouth, I ran my tongue over the wound, felt and tasted the blood where my teeth had cut through the lip, but it was so cold out, I didn't feel the pain. So my friend picked up the sled and we headed for home. Oh, no! I thought. Ma will be wild!

"What were you doing? Where were you?? Here, put this ice cube on your lip! Now you stay in the house! No more sledding today! What were you doing on Rotundi's hill anyway? You're too small to sled over there. It's too big a hill for you! You need to stay closer to home!" As I sat there nursing my puffed up sore lip, I was doggedly planning to go back to that beautiful hill the next day. I lOVED the Winter! I lOVED the cold! I LOVED the fun and excitement of a fast ride on my sled down that forbidden hill!

Summer on Cottage Street

The Elliotts lived next door. In the far corner of their yard, the summer grass was as tall as my legs were long. There was a stone fireplace in the mowed area where Mr. Elliott would burn stuff. I liked the tall grass in the un-mowed part and the quietness of being all alone there. It was always an adventure, walking alone in the warmth of the tall summer grass. Alone until the Grasshopper appeared–deep in the openness, close to the earth, all green and still–poised majestically on a leaf. I crouched down on my knees and got very close to him until I saw every tiny bit of his bright green self–his body long and full with lots of pretty green legs, each one bent like a knee. I was very close and very still and the moment has lasted a whole lifetime! Why?

Because I remember it.

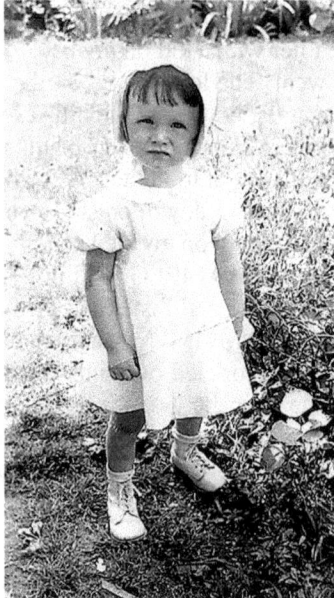

Barbara age 5

When I was five I climbed the small apple tree in the Elliott's yard that I had been told not to climb because the tree was too small. I climbed it anyway and one day, I slipped and slid down the tree trunk until my thigh caught on a small sharp broken branch. The branch ripped deeply into my flesh causing a gush of red blood. My disobedience frightened me more than the sight of the blood. I had been told not to and I did. And now I was hurt and had to go home and explain. Earlier that day, I had noticed a broken milk bottle next to the Elliott's back steps. A convenient lie right in front of me, I could easily tell and get away with it. So I went home and said I fell on the broken milk bottle near Mrs. Elliott's back steps. I still have the white scar tissue on my left thigh. It was the lessor of two evils to lie rather than face the rage and accusations and finger pointing that made my stomach hurt.

Fall on Cottage Street

Tommy Elliott, next door, was born a year before I was born in August. He was the only boy in his family and the youngest and although he was more of a boy's boy and was usually off playing with the boys, we hung around as pals sometimes. His sister Eileen was the oldest child and she became a Sister of Providence when she grew up. Doris was second and Connie was three years old when Tommy was born. Tommy had a wide smile and large, vacant brown eyes that always stared straight ahead.

It was mid-September. I was seven and Tommy was eight and we went far from home to play in the tall grass near Sweet Water Brook in the shallow woods off Lindenwood Road near the train tracks. That is where I met Tommy's friend, 10 year old Timmy Kimbal. Tommy left early to help another boy do his paper route and left me with Timmy who taught me some new games to play. They were naked games and we did things we were not supposed to do. When it was over, I ran home with excitement, but by the time I got there I was filled with much shame and feelings of loneliness. I was scared, like I was betraying everyone–did not quite know why, but told no one. And I kept going back for more. And by the time I was nine, more kids played in the woods near the brook–kids from other streets. I didn't know how to stop. I was trapped in deceit and shame with this immense secret. I felt myself shrinking, deeper and deeper inside a kind of barbed wire life.

I did not know it at the time, but polio was just around the corner.

And I didn't know this either,

I was... glad, when Polio finally rescued me!

Ma

One summer afternoon I found Ma sitting on the edge of her bed. Her room was dark. The shades were down to keep out the hot afternoon sun. Their bedroom faced west and got the heat of summer.

She was looking at a small mahogany jewelry box that had a red velvet lining and little shelves and drawers, containing green, red, amber and purple gem stones. When I asked what they were, she said "Old treasure Gifts from Joe." I sat on the bed across from her as she dreamed out loud–telling me stories about each item. She held up a string of crystal beads and said she liked to wear the beads on black velvet–that they were a gift that Joe brought her from an exotic trip to a foreign port. She said Joe was a Merchant Marine.

I'm not sure how old I was at the time, but she must have thought not old enough to understand much of what she was saying, although she made me cross my heart and promise. "Don't ever tell your father. Your father is a good man. A good father, but Joe... Joe is the man I really loved. These are all gifts from Joe. He brought me gifts from all over the world." And she would drift far away, remembering things and caressing each piece. There were several afternoons like that one. When she was done, she would place the box in her bureau drawer under some scarves.

"Marry the man who'll be with you," Ma quoted Nana when she would read about or hear about a local romance turned sour. In later years, Ma stopped worrying about how much I understood and told me a lot more. How Joe desperately wanted to be with her. He tried, by quitting the Merchant Marines and taking a job at the GE, but only for a short while.

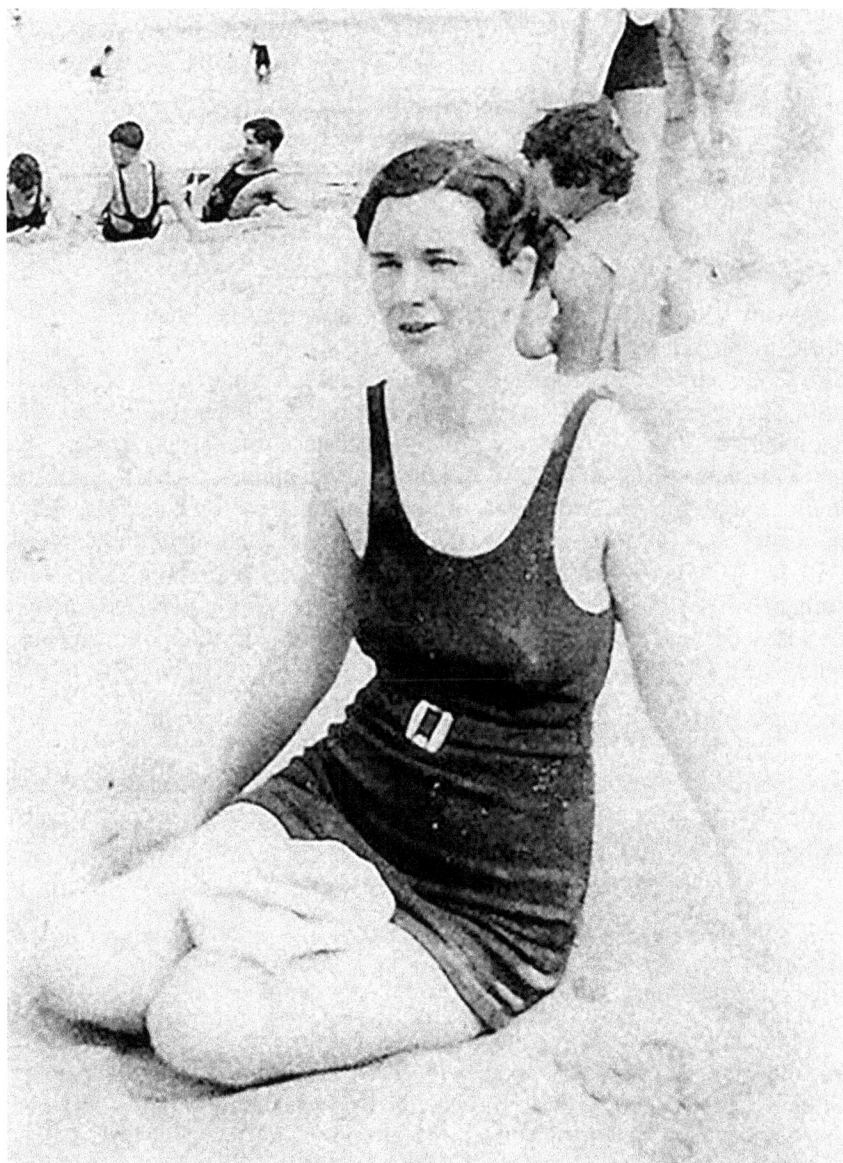

Ma

He just couldn't be happy on dry land for any length of time and finally went back to Sea. again, for good. Years later, Etta, Joe's sister, told Ma that

Joe threw all her letters overboard. And even hearing that, she never stopped loving him.

"Joe was a red head. He had red curly hair. He came from Fitchburg." "His mother's name was Delia" Ma told me one afternoon as she unfolded a silk kimono from China, then folded it back up again and lovingly replaced it under some delicate clothing in the bureau drawer with the secret warning not to tell Dad. Those were rare quiet, sad and intimate moments that I had with Ma.

Many years later, when she was in her 80's, and Dad had passed. We drove to Fitchburg and Ma found the house she remembered on Boylston Street. We parked across from the house and after a while we saw a car pull up and an elderly man and woman got out and went into the house. It was Joe and his sister Etta. Ma suddenly had the enthusiasm of a teenager. Dare she go to the door? Ring the bell? While she was deciding, Joe came out of the house and began walking down the sidewalk across from us. Ma didn't hesitate. She opened the car door, crossed the street and caught up with him. "Hi, Joe." she said. For a moment or two Joe was taken aback, but soon recognized her. "My, my, where did you come from?" He took her arm and they walked back to the house. She said hello to Etta and both of them came out to the car to meet me. Joe was caught up in memories.

He went back in the house and brought out a picture album. He said, "I was a Merchant Marine." Yes, I know, I thought. There were photos of the woman he had married and their children. She bore him three sons but she died when the youngest was nine. Etta raised the children while Joe remained at Sea.

It was quite a day. But Ma never saw Joe again. They sent cards at Christmas and on their birthdays. From that day onward, she was comfortable in knowing that she had made the right decision. Nana was right. She had married the man who would "be with her".

Ma could best be described as stoical in her demeanor–a deep believer and devoted church goer. She loved Our Lady's Sodality and served as Prefect one year. She was proud of her leadership ability and her association with Father Coakley, the group's spiritual director. Father Coakley loved the meetings held in the lady's homes and especially loved the special homemade desserts the ladies served with tea. Her Presentation made her grateful she had been born a Catholic. Her faith sustained her when she didn't let anything or anyone else close enough to help. She held on for dear life to her devotion to the Sacred Heart of Jesus, to Mary the Mother of God and to St. Joseph, the Patron saint of the worker. Her faith kept Ma strong.

Ma's Sewing Club met regularly in each other's homes, too. Ma and Aunt Dot (Flynn) Mary Gilmartin, Wini Russell and her sister, Laura Rivers, Molly Ahern and Helen McCarthy. Ma took great pride in those opportunities to shine and shine she did! She sparkled at her dining room table, surrounded by her china tea cups, crystal dessert "stem ware," linen napkins and lace table cloth. Her friends raved over her cooking!

Dad

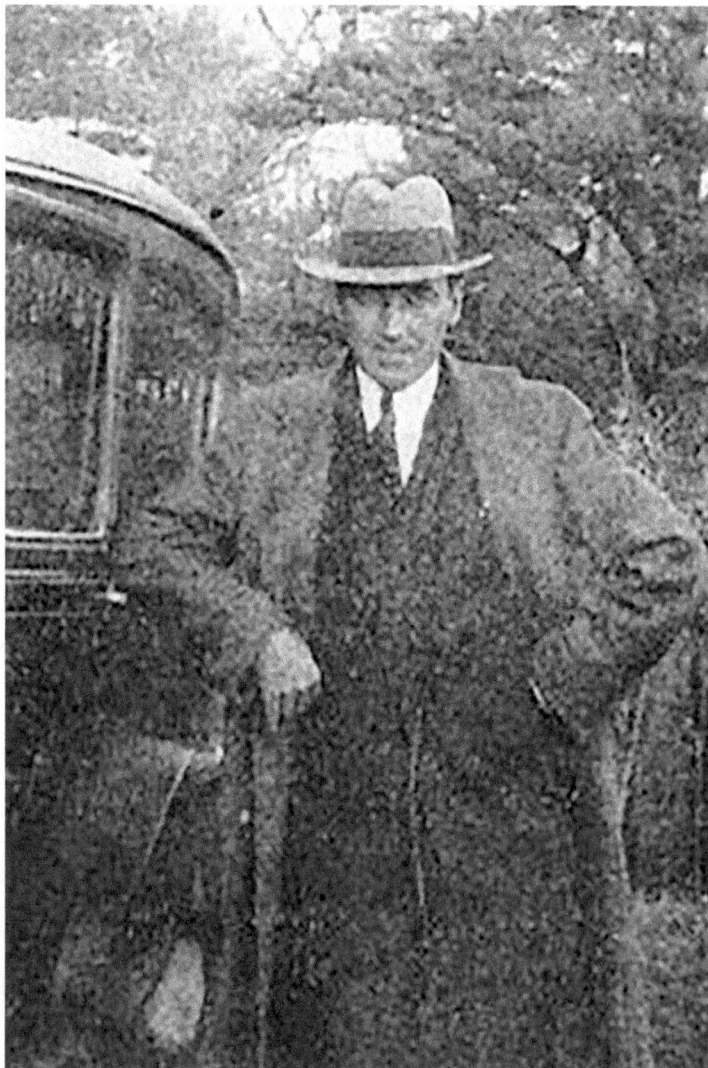

"James, Joseph, Henry, Wendell, Vincent, David, Bancroft Duffy." That's what Dad would say when I touched my finger tip to his chin and asked him teasingly "What's your name?" And he'd say, "James, Joseph, Henry, Wendell, Vincent, David, Bancroft Duffy." "No, Sir." I'd say. "Your name is Henry James Duffy and sometimes Harry." Ma called Dad Harry. So did Aunt Dot, Uncle Jack, Aunt Nora, all of the McAuliffe's and everyone else who knew Dad's family. Dad's friends at work all called him Henry, But it amused him to play the pretend name game with me and become "James, Joseph, Henry, Wendell, Vincent, David, Bancroft Duffy."

Harry, my father, was a gentle man. He smoked a pipe, wore Khaki pants and shirt (workingman's style) and liked to walk around the house in his stocking feet. He would take pictures of us anytime at all. We didn't have to be dressed up for Dad to take our picture. He had a Dark Room with a soft red bulb down in the cellar, where he developed his pictures. He'd sit on a tall stool and stir the strong smelling solution over the slowly developing pictures with a long glass stirrer. Then he would string the wet pictures up to dry with clothes pins along a line strung over his work bench.

Dad was quiet and easy to be with. He liked to work in the garden and mow the lawn. He liked to shovel the snow. And Dad liked me. He liked to have me around. He never said, "Go away." Or "I'm too busy for you." He would say, "Come on with me Stevie. You and I will stick together." Of course, I could speculate today why he called me Stevie, but that never dawned on me. I just liked how it felt when he did call me that, because it was a continual reminder that Dad really liked me.

Dad and I spent many summer days and hours in the woods of Georgetown. The old road was overgrown with weeds and the car couldn't clear the underbrush, so we would walk into Camp Peewee from the road, carrying silver pails to collect blueberries. Camp Peewee was Dad's nickname for a tar paper shack the size of a one car garage set deep in the woods near the pond. Our cousins, the McAuliffes, owned the land around Camp Peewee. Sometimes my cousin Jackie Flynn would come with us to pick blueberries, or Uncle "Flo" McAuliffe would come along with his kids, Johnny and Joanie. But I liked it best when I was eight and nine and ten and it was just Dad and me. That's how I like to remember those days. Dad would pack a lunch that he made himself–usually peanut butter and jelly sandwiches and a thermos full of lemonade. We ate by the car before heading into the bushes to gather the blueberries. Dad taught me to pick the berries one at a time. He said we should pick the berries carefully, respectfully. "It's the outing out here in these fine woods that's most important," he would say and I thought so too. Being together in the lovely quiet woods, picking the berries and bringing them home to Ma. After Dad cleaned them Ma would put them up in preserve jars and we would have fresh and delectable blueberry pies all Winter. Ma didn't need any help making her pies and didn't want any distractions. She chose to be isolated for her part of it–not willing or wanting to share herself or her tasks with the rest of us, like Dad did. Dad preferred to have company along–me, Paul, or Peggy. It was okay to be with him when he developed the pictures or while he worked in the garden. Paul would sit with Dad in his leather chair while he read The Evening Globe and smoked his pipe, until Paul got too tall– too big to fit and he had to give up that snug place where he felt so warm and safe. I have missed so much my outings with Dad. And, like Paul, I miss that safe place by his side.

Dad was proud of the house he had built on Cottage Street in Stoneham Massachusetts in 1935. And he was proud of the job he held all through The Depression and the money he and Ma were able to save in the Cooperative Bank. And Ma too was proud of her job as a stenographer in Boston that she held during those years when so many others were out of work and had little or no money. They considered themselves extremely fortunate and in respect for that, made careful and discriminating choices when it came time to be married and plan their future. They hired Mr. Bears, a builder who didn't have much work because of the Depression and told him the kind of house they wanted him to build. The house lot they chose was between two bungalows. The Elliots on one side and the Lockharts on the other. Ma and Dad preferred the Cape style with the bedrooms and the bath upstairs. They insisted that it be modeled after Helen and Jim Worden's Cape on Royal Street that Mr. Bears had built a few years earlier. The land and the house cost $4,500.00 in 1935. Ma and Dad were proud to say they had the house fully furnished and half paid for when they moved in on June 10th 1935. Ma loved to talk about her prized bedroom set, custom built with rich, dark inlaid mahogany twin beds, Ma's dresser and Dad's Chifferobe, with an inside mirror, shelf, bar and key. Each room was furnished and attractively adorned in light of Ma's good taste for color and style. Keeping the house dusted and polished and sparkling was her joy.

The house was set high on the sloping side of a small hill, which leveled off at the top and toward the rear, which Dad immediately perceived to be a fine place for his flowers and vegetables–just the right amount of sun and shade. The front of the house was encased in a stone foundation with a garage underneath the front porch. A half dozen cement stairs led from the sidewalk to the ten wooden stairs above which climbed to the porch.

Dad loved the screened in front porch, where he could sit comfortably in the spring and summertime, enjoying his pipe and newspaper and looking down on cars and passer byes and other goings on in the neighborhood; as much as Ma loved her dining room and they both loved the fireplace in the living room. Ma was the only one in her crowd to have a house of her own and Dad was equally pleased to own his own place. They both liked company. Ma invited her friends from Lynn and Dad's friends from work would visit on Saturday nights and listen to the ball game over the Philco Console radio in the living room. On Sundays, Ma liked to cook a special desert and serve her guests in the dining room using her best china plates and sterling silver tea spoons. Her crystal candle stick holders were on either side of the crystal bowl in the center of the lace covered dining room table. The chandelier cast a soft light over Ma's lovely spread.

Of course, all of that would be rudely and permanently altered when Polio arrived and Ma's cherished showpiece dining room set had to be replaced with the huge hospital bed, a wheelchair, plaster night casts, bed pans, sandbags, splints and blow bottles–essentially a full time bed, bath, living room, library and eatery for yours truly.

"The Gov'ner." That's how Dad referred to his father, Jim Duffy. I never knew Dad's parents. I only know the stories I heard from Ma and Dad–mostly Ma. Dad visited the graves of the Gov'ner and his mother, Margaret at St Patrick's Cemetery in Stoneham every Memorial Day. I would go with him and watch him deposit a red geranium on his Dad's grave and a basket of flowers on Margaret's, who was the first to be buried in our family plot. Dad's been there now since 1975 and Ma since 1992. Next door the Flynns have their plot, where my Aunt (Dad's sister Dorothy) and Uncle Jack Flynn rest as well.

There is room for one more full body or two cremated ones in our plot. Who will it be? Peggy? Paul? Or (being a priest) Paul might be buried with the Maryknoll fathers. Maybe I'll be there with the love of my life, my dear Mary, as I am now with her during life. Or Peggy with Ma and Dad. Peggy talks about being cremated. She asks me if I am going to be cremated. "We'd both fit in that way," she said, curiously belonging and making room. But, for me...? What about Mary? I like the idea of being with Mary better.

Most of what I know about Dad's family life I heard from Ma. And she got her stories, not from Dad, but from Aunt Dot (Flynn) and the McAuliffe's. Margaret (Murphy) Duffy was the strongest one. She was born in Salem, Massachusetts and Aunt Nora was her sister. Margaret was a childless widow when she met and married Jim Duffy in the mid 1890's. She was a nurse–not by education but by practice. She assisted at home births and took care of the sick in their homes. She had two children by Jim. Dad (Henry James) was born in 1899 and eleven months later Aunt Dot was born. They were born in Chelsea, where Jim had a barber shop. Problem was, Jim was a binge drinker. Every few months he'd go off and be gone for days. Eventually his drinking caused him to lose the barber shop and eventually his marriage and his family. Ma Duffy didn't have much patience with Jim and gave him his walking papers. A separation they called it. Not a divorce. I don't know where he went or what he did. But he died on the Feast of the Immaculate Conception, on December 8th, when Dad was in his twenties. Jim was sixty-eight when on his way home from Mass, he dropped dead in the street of a heart attack with his Rosary Beads in his hand. Dad told me the Gov'ner had read the Bible three times, all the way through.

The Chelsea fire in 1908 destroyed Dad's home and for a year, when he was nine, he lived with his cousins, Phil, Flo and Mammie, McAuliffe in Wakefield. Dad was in third grade that year and attended classes at the Westward School–a small one room school house in the Park Section of Wakefield on the hill on Prospect Street. The little red school house is still on Prospect Street and is still an active elementary school. Dad's roots and fondest memories were really there in Wakefield with the McAuliffes–Phil, Flo, young Mammie, Aunt Mammie and Uncle Tim. They lived on North Ave, across the street from Lake Quannipowitt, and even after moving back with his mother and sister Dorothy in Chelsea, Dad grew up spending all his summers and weekends in Wakefield. His life centered around activity on the lake. Dad's memories were stories of boyhood adventures on the lake– swimming, fishing and skating. When he was twelve Dad broke his arm early in the summer and the day the cast came off he was so enthused to have his arm back he swam the 300 yards from the boat house to the top of the lake. When Aunt Mammie found out she went wild on him!

The Rifle Range, later known as Camp Curtis Guild, a National Guard Camp, was at the North end of the lake where Dad, Phil and Flo got jobs marking targets for target practice in the summer. In Winter they got jobs at the Ice House which was also at the head of the lake. Also, fishing was a year round activity that they enjoyed together throughout their younger and retirement years and in the Fall they indulged their love of duck hunting. Dad loved the changing seasons all of his life and enjoyed the activities each season brought forth.

Dad and his cousins were life long friends. Like brothers, Ma said.

Dad and "the Doc" Phil, were often mistaken for each other because of their similar sharp features and expressive blue eyes, but Dad felt the most closeness to Flo who was a school teacher and had a deep appreciation of

Nature and Literature. Dad was disappointed that he missed enlisting in WWI because he was too young. His cousins Phil and Flo didn't go in either because they were in college. Dad was the youngest of the three.

Later in life, Dad and Flo went to the lake every day to feed the wild ducks. The middle years of their lives were different. They had different opportunities. Phil, Flo and Mammie all went to college–Tufts, BC and Emerson. Aunt Mammie saw to that Phil enrolled in Tufts Dental School and became a dentist. Flo had a Master's Degree and was a school principal. Mammie died of TB at twenty-eight, after completing Emerson College. Uncle Tim was a Janitor at the Parker House in Boston and Dad never knew how they got the money to send their children to college.

Flo taught in Dorchester and married Marie who was a Latin teacher.

All summer, every summer they left for Camp Theodore Roosevelt on Pleasant Lake in Island Falls, Maine as soon as school closed and they returned the day after Labor Day. Flo started out there as a camp counselor when he was a college student and eventually bought the cottages–all eight of them as well as the field house and he added two log cabins. Ma and Dad spent their Honeymoon at Pleasant Lake and from that time on, Flo called their cabin *The Honeymoon Cabin.*

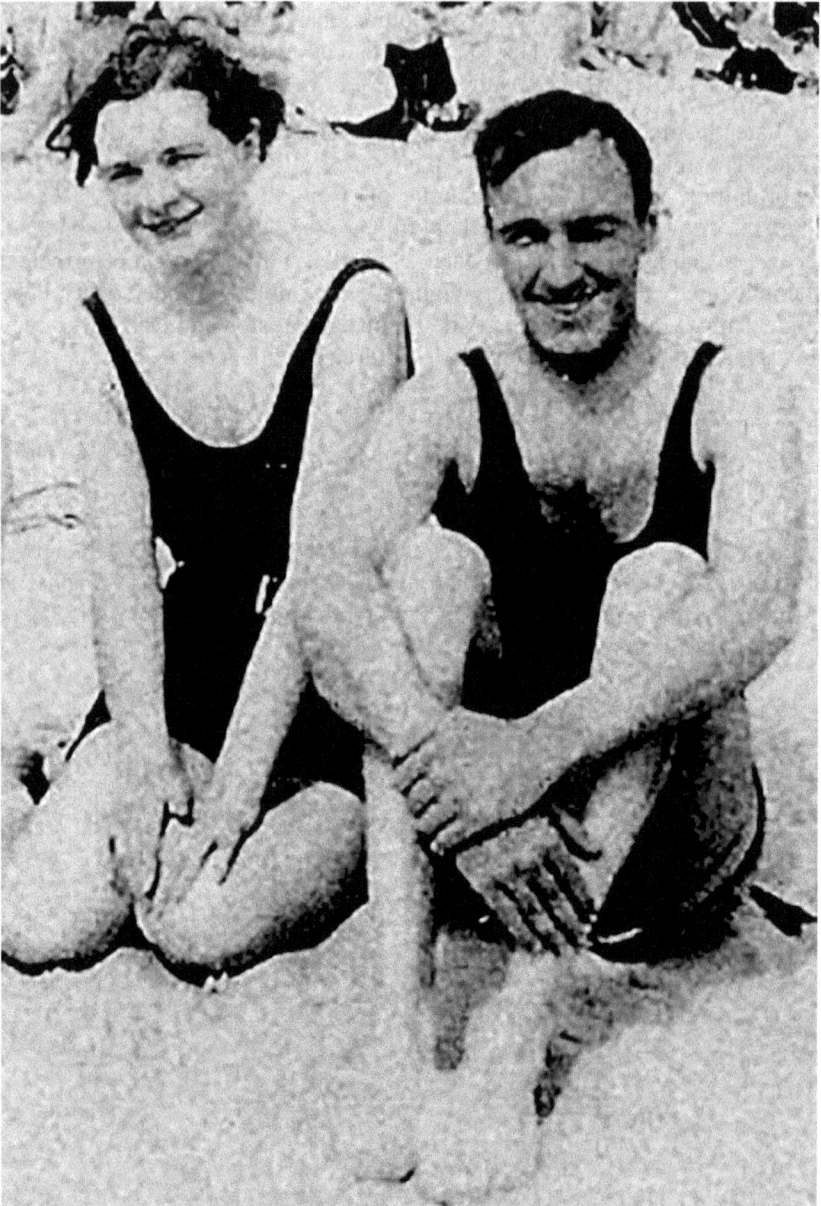

The Honeymooners

Dad had to quit school in the eighth grade to help support his mother and Aunt Dot. He got his first job at the Chelsea Clock Factory. He had no shoes to wear on his first day on the job, so with his mother's permission, he peeled the heels off a pair of her shoes and wore them. Later, after he got his license to drive, he got a job working for Mrs. French in Wakefield, driving her car for her. He liked to talk about that job.

When Mr. French died and was cremated, Dad had to drive his ashes home. He said he didn't know what to say to him, so he hummed "Anchors Away". He continued to drive Mrs. French around until he turned twenty-one and got a job at the Malden Electric Company as a Meter Reader. He retired from the Electric Company forty-four years later when he was sixty-five. Most of those years on the job he was a cable splicer, working with men who were bigger and seemingly stronger than he, but nonetheless Dad was able to handle the large cables right along with the best of them. He never complained and I never knew him to take a day off. He went out in snowstorms and hurricanes when the lines went down and the power went out. He worked a lot of overtime. Dad was proud of his steady, reliable job that paid good wages and offered excellent benefits. He was a Union Man and took good care of his family. We grew up thinking that the McAuliffe's were Dad's real family and we visited Aunt Mammie and Uncle Tim on Saturdays. I trudged along close to Dad's side among the chickens, hens, ducks and geese Uncle Tim raised in the back yard.

Dad's mother died in December of 1935–the same year Dad and Ma were married. She was only sick for a week–had an ulcer on the side of her leg and suddenly one night she died. She was waked at Aunt Dot's house where she lived. Ma told the story of how on the night of the wake, during the Rosary, Nana fell asleep and began to snore loudly, embarrassing Ma to death! Ma said it was a good thing Margaret died, because she was very bossy and would run Dad's household the way she ran Aunt Dot's. Strong willed and opinionated, she would bring her friends over and say to Ma, "Come on, Suzie girl, put the coffee on and let's play cards." Ma said it was Ma Duffy who directed the building of the house she and Dad had built. It was Ma Duffy who said where the electrical outlets needed to go. Ma resented and liked her at the same time. Aunt Dot was dominated by her just as Dad had been and another part of her legacy was that she cheated at cards.

Of the three cousins, Dad was the first to die at seventy-six. He died of Congestive Heart Failure at home with Ma, Paul, me and Peggy close by. Phil was next at eighty-five. He practiced Dentistry until the day he died of Heart Failure. Flo out lived them all. He died when he was ninety in his chair in the kitchen. When Dad died, Flo said "Now I won't have anyone to tell things to." They were friends all the way to the end. When they went duck hunting Dad would bring his camera and take beautiful pictures of the sunrise over Indian River–their special section of the Merrimac. Later he put all his slides together and he and Phil gave slide shows and talked about their experiences. They also liked to pick blueberries and cranberries. Dad would get mad at Phil from time to time and with Flo, too, but his displeasure didn't last. They cared a lot for each other and never had a real falling out. In other words, they never were not friends.

Later on in her life, Ma often said that Dad had a good life. I think maybe she envied him. She would often comment on Dad's hobbies–his garden, his photography, his love of nature and his friendship with the McAuliffes–a life Ma didn't share, really. But they both basically believed in what were the two most important things in their lives–family and the Catholic Church. They were good citizens and they made a home for their three children.

The New Baby

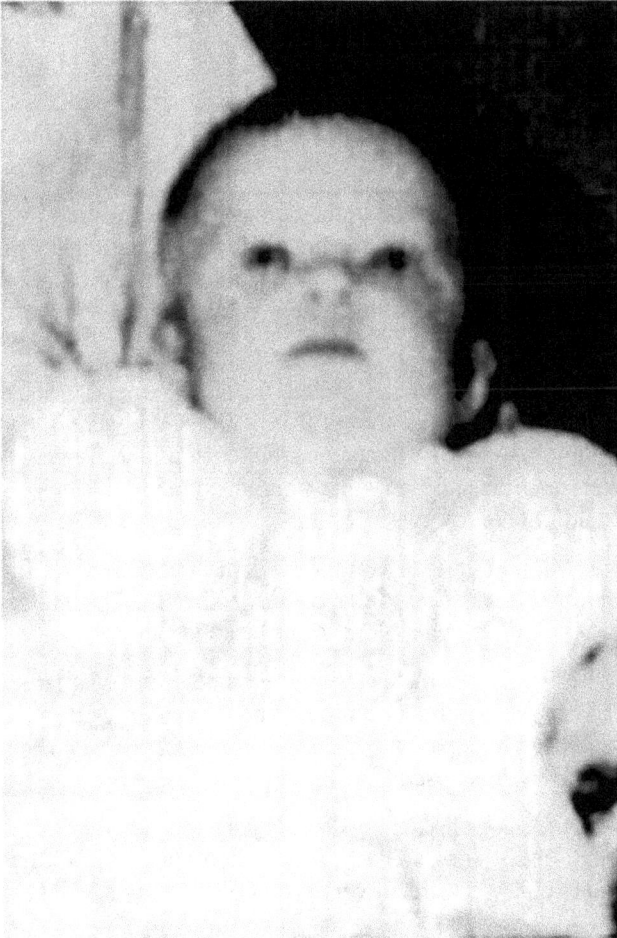

Paul Joseph Duffy

49

I was seven when Ma told me that we were going to have a baby! We were in the kitchen and Ma invited me to sit on her lap as she confided the news. It's a secret, she said and I asked if Dad knew. She said yes he did and Peggy knew. And Aunt Dot? Yes, she knew, too. What about cousins Bette Jean and Jackie? Did they know? No, not yet. Later, when Bette Jean heard the news she wanted her mother, Aunt Dot, to have a baby, too. But this was very, very special; no one I knew had a brand new baby!

Just before the baby arrived, Ma's Sewing Club friends had a baby shower for her. The Shower was at Wini Russell's house with Laura Rivers, Helen McCarthy, Molly Ahern, Mary Gilmartin, Aunt Dot and Ma's friends from Our Lady's Sodality. I was super excited. It was better than Christmas! There were blue satin shoes, a white knitted sweater and bonnet, a round clear plastic ball with multicolored tiny toys inside for the baby's bath. I cherished those little gifts in anticipation of our new baby that I hoped would be a boy.

On April 15, 1947 Ma stood in the doorway of our bedroom and told me and Peggy that she was going to the hospital to have the baby. It was late in the night and Ma had on her black seal skin coat. I became super excited the next day when Dad told us we had a new baby brother who weighed seven pounds and fourteen ounces!

The day Ma and the baby came home from the Winchester Hospital, Dad picked up Peggy and me from school at noontime. We were in the back seat when Ma got into the car with the baby over her shoulder. He was all wrapped up in blankets and he had the white knitted bonnet on that Ma got at the shower. I couldn't take my eyes off him!

At home, Ma laid the baby on the kitchen table where we finally had a good look at him. He was beautiful and admired by all the neighbors, relatives and friends–Mrs. Elliott, Aunt Nora, Aunt Dot and Bette Jean!

It was a very special time! A few weeks later Aunt Margaret and Uncle Sid arrived. They weren't really our aunt and uncle, but were Ma's very best friends who became Godparents of our baby when he was chris-tened at St. Patrick's church as *Paul Joseph*.

Paul wore the same christening dress Nana had made for Ma's christening in 1905. Peggy and I had also worn it, so when Paul wore it, the dress was over forty years old. We were all very proud of our very special baby boy!

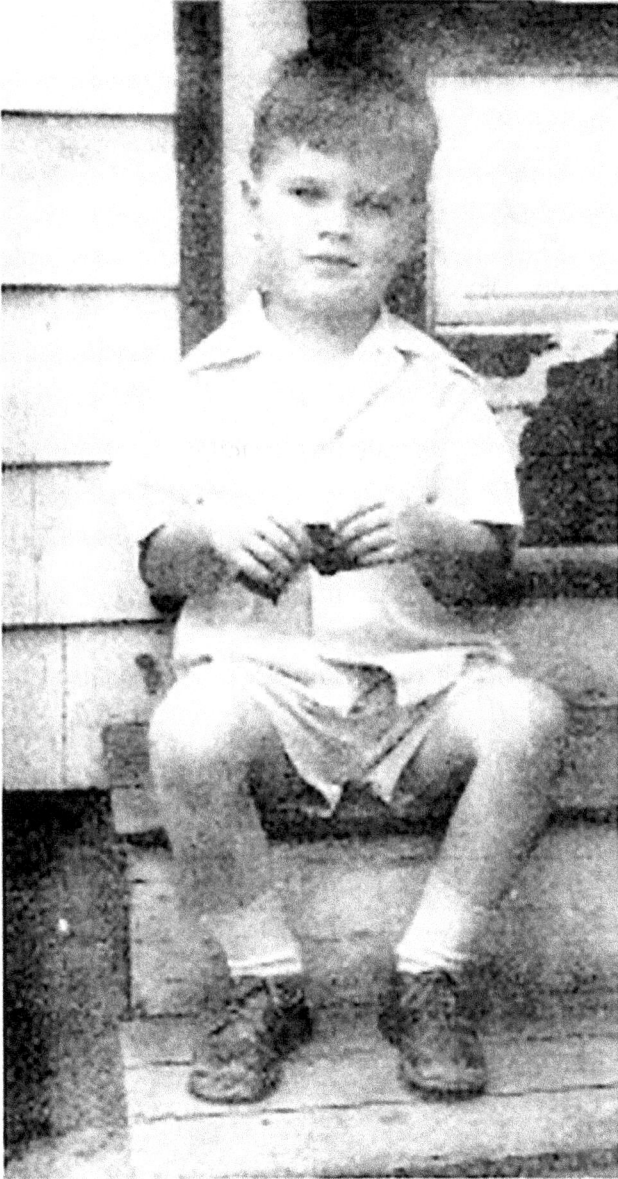

Paul

I remember the day that we lost Paul. It was hot and sunny. I was nine, Paul was two and we couldn't find him anywhere. He wasn't in front of the house on the porch, on the sidewalk, or out in the street. He wasn't sitting in the shade of the back steps which he liked to do in the summer heat and he was nowhere in the yard, or in the deep grass that bordered the back lawn and the railroad tracks. I ran through the Elliott's back yard, pushing and ducking the clothes and sheets that hung from her clothes line on my way to Gusterferro's house up the street.

Suddenly the whistle of an oncoming freight train struck a deep flash of terror through me. Thinking he might have wandered onto the tracks, my heart pounded like it was the only organ in my body. As the train thundered by, I pressed my hands over my eyes and felt such glorious relief when I dared to pluck my palms away and didn't see his body smashed in pieces on the tracks. I glanced toward our yard and caught a glimpse of Ma rushing toward our house and raced after her. I followed her in the back door, through the kitchen and upstairs.

The fading whistle of the freight train echoed through the open screened window in the bedroom. I clung to Ma's apron as she and I gazed with unspoken relief at our baby Paul, blissfully cradled in deep sleep in his crib (sides up).

I loved my little brother Paul. I especially liked him when he was two years old. His light brown skin was silky-soft and he had dimples on the back of his hands. He was chubby and agreeable and fit neatly into my doll carriage. I would push him round and round through the house–through the living room, the dining room and kitchen, round and round. I loved to hold his hand and walk along with him. When Peggy was mean, I would protect him–shield him with my arms and shoulders. Protecting him from Peggy overcame some of my feelings of fear and that made me love him even more. One day I overheard Ma talking to Mrs. Gallella. She said "Barbara can't take care of Paul. She doesn't know how and she's too small." I was crushed when I heard those words, because I loved Paul and I took very good care of him. It was sad, but Ma didn't see me as capable even way back then–even when I knew I was.

Ma didn't encourage me–even as she doesn't now. It is a bit ridiculous. Here I am, fifty-one years of age and Ma tells me I'm a good girl when I clear the table or make my bed. She tells Paul he's a good boy. Three good children, she says.

Ma would feel terribly threatened if she saw her children as the capable adults we are today. She'd lose control. Her heart was pure, although she scolded as quickly as she praised.

Plum Island With the Flynns

In the summer of 1946 we spent a week at Plum Island. Paul hadn't been born yet. Jackie and I were seven that year and Peggy and Bette Jean were ten. Aunt Dot and Uncle Jack had a cottage for two weeks and they invited us to share the cottage with them for the second week. The cottage wasn't far from the water where the waves were really active and we were cautioned over and over about the dangerous undertow. We would run the few hundred yards to the beach and the black hot top burned as I hopped quickly from foot to foot. Jackie didn't mind. He was tough and his body was lean and strong. I followed close behind him to the water's edge where he stood on the sandy beach and scaled small flat stones way out into the water.

The tuna boats came in to dock nearby where the fishermen had scales big enough to weigh the massive tunas that were hung up in rows allowing the onlookers to see and admire. Basically, it was a working beach filled with fishermen coming in with their catches, while seagulls cawed and nipped at each other as they waited overhead to swoop down and eat up the unwanted remnants of the days catch. The clams were stored in bins of salt water inside a huge wooden building and we kids would dash through the building, grab fistfuls of clams out of the water and squirt them at each other.

A pier and swimming beach for the residents was a little further down the shore. Jackie and I were not allowed to go in the water alone, but we were allowed to sit on the pier with a fishing line and catch flounders.

Peggy and Bette Jean were also there with Billy Flynn–Jackie and Bette's half–brother, recently returned from the War in Europe where he had been awarded the Distinguished Flying Cross as a B-17 Pilot. Billy was Uncle Jack's grown up son by his first marriage to Mammie McAuliffe–Aunt Dot and Dad's first cousin. Mammie died in her late twenties of TB when Billy was only six. And a few years later, Aunt Dot married Mammie's widower, Jack Flynn. As a child and growing up through his teen years, Billy continued to live with his Grandmother over in Wakefield and occasionally would spend time with his father, like that time at Plum Island. Billy took us to Newburyport on a day that was rainy and cold and not a good beach day. We went to the Arcade and then to a movie. Billy picked me up and put me on his shoulders. I had fun that day. Aunt Dot stayed home and cooked all the meals and Ma, pregnant with Paul, stayed with her. Dad spent a lot of time on the beach with us. I would watch him swim from the shore. He made it look so easy. He didn't swim straight out. He swam across the water. And he told us to do the same thing, because the safest way to swim was to not go way out over our heads. Uncle Jack, not a swimmer, enjoyed his vacation time on the cottage porch sipping cold beer and observing the neighbors. Everything was casual and everyone dressed casually on that friendly and wholesome Plum Island retreat. Uncle Jack had a joke that he never tired of playing on his male visitors. He had a beer mug full of wax–the golden color of beer. He would keep the mug icy-cold in the fridge and when a beer drinking male friend or relative would drop by on weekends, Uncle Jack would put real beer foam on top and hand the fake beer to him, which he would anticipate with great relish in the summer heat. As his guest lifted it greedily to his lips, his nose would smush through the foam and jam against the hard wax. The surprise looks and frowns on his face were hilarious to witness.

Aunt Dot was always kind and ready with a hug or a wet face-cloth to wash away tears when kids feelings were hurt. And she made fudge. There was sand all around the outside of the cottage and I can still feel that hot sand beneath my feet squishing between my toes. My mind often travels back to that week in Plum Island where I am always seven, always feeling the sand under my feet, awed by Jackie's energy and athleticism and comforted by Dad's gentle pipe smoking presence.

Aunt Dot and Uncle Jack's marriage was like Ma and Dad's marriage. A mutually agreed upon arrangement. They slept in twin beds, too. Their marriage was a way to have a home and a family. A way to get on in life with passion left behind in other relationships, ended by death or poor decisions. Theirs were loveless marriages, cold and distant, without visible signs of affection between them. Aunt Dot never got over the love of her life, Ernie, a master electrician who was electrocuted on the job six weeks before they were to be married. As time went on Aunt Dot married Uncle Jack and gave birth to Bette Jean in 1936 and Jackie in 1939. She did her best to suppress her memory of Ernie and devoted herself to Bette Jean. Curling her hair and selecting the proper clothes and insisting on proper behavior. She would hover by her daughter as she practiced the piano, constantly giving her instruction and criticism–carefully and intensely grooming her to stand out physically and musically at the periodic recitals, dreaming that one day she would be a concert pianist at Carnegie Hall. She had another dream that Bette Jean did fulfill. She grew up to be Queen of the Winter Carnival Ball in her Senior year at Stoneham High School. Peggy was one of her Attendants. Bette Jean later married Peter Berrini, who was captain of the football team and

King of that same Carnival Ball and the very boy Aunt Dot had picked out for Bette Jean when they were in sixth grade at the North School. Many years after Peter and Bette were married and had spawned three daughters, Peter looked straight at his self-satisfying spouse one day and said, "I want a divorce." I have always admired Peter for that. It was like he woke up one morning and said "I'm out of this fairy tale."

Peggy got in the way of Ma's devotion to her memories, similar to the way Jackie would barge in and interfere with Aunt Dot's vicarious fantasies, which when weren't interrupted, allowed her to forget about Ernie.

Bette Jean had no life of her own until Aunt Dot died, when Bette Jean was forty-six years old. While Aunt Dot was alive, Bette Jean was a pretend person living in Aunt Dot's imagination. After she passed, Bette became more real and married her friend, Charlie, who was utterly devoted to her and they have made a fine, happy life together, since.

Jackie's way of surviving Aunt Dot's obsession with Bette Jean was to be rebellious, obnoxious, oppositional and confrontational. He showed the world that all was not well in that house–the way Peggy showed the world that all was not well in our house. No one seemed to understand the meaning behind their anger. No one wanted to understand. So Jackie became the scapegoat in his family the way Peggy became the scapegoat in our family. Jackie got the short end of the stick from Aunt Dot and the violent end of Uncle Jack's belt. Peggy caught Ma's anger and Dad's rejection.

Aunt Dot's and Uncle Jack's House

There was a huge oak tree sixty or seventy feet high in the back lawn of Aunt Dot and Uncle Jack's house at 25 Oak Street and its branches spread out, covering the entire back lawn and the two car garage that stood at the end of the long driveway between the two, eight room, brown shingled houses owned by the two brothers, Tom and Jack Flynn and built by their father, Edward Flynn. The seven acres of land bordering the houses on Oak Street was part of the old Flynn family homestead that still borders where the south side of the field used to be. Now there are twenty-seven houses, where there was once seven acres of rich farmland, known as *Flynn's Field*. Uncle Tom raised pigs in one corner of the field and each spring *Murphy's Farm* leased sections to plant potatoes and corn, leaving plenty of room to gather hay for their animals and room for the boy's baseball diamond, which was Jackie's main interest, except when he needed to hide out in the cornfield to escape his raging Father's flailing leather belt.

Twenty-five Oak Street was not far from our house at 37 Cottage Street. You went left on William Street, around the corner, up Elm to Oak and down Oak to number 25 and there you were, four minutes later, at Aunt Dot's back door.

Dad visited his sister Dot whenever he felt like it and Aunt Dot was always ready with a cup of tea, a friendly smile and the latest gossip for him. Often Dad took me along. Jackie was free to run off and do as he pleased and I would race off after him. Uncle Jack Flynn was an auto mechanic, but for a while he leased and managed a car dealership, until the war came along and he could no longer get the parts or the cars to sell and he lost it all. He was back working as a mechanic for someone else again, which he especially despised. He worked long hours, six days a week and was not home much. He would come home at unpredictable hours and Aunt Dot often cooked meals for him late at night. He liked company at Christmas and when he drank he was jolly and everyone had a good time.

Uncle Jack and Uncle Tom, would listen to the Red Sox and Boston Braves baseball games on Summer Sundays, as they drank beer and smoked cigarettes under the welcoming shade of the Great Oak, which was known as the most perfectly shaped tree (without pruning) in the town Of Stoneham,

Massachusetts. Uncle Jack usually had a car parked on the lawn waiting for mechanical repairs. And the Iceman would drive his truck into the long driveway and stop in front of the garage. He would grab his cruel looking metal tongs from the back of the truck, clamp onto a cumbersome chunk of ice, hoist it over his shoulder onto his rubber protective shield and head up the walk toward the back door where Aunt Dot would be waiting to greet him. She held open the screen door as he entered the back hall where the wooden ice chest stood ready to receive the 24 inch square chunk of ice. I was fascinated by much of Aunt Dot's house that was so different from ours. We had a refrigerator in our back hall, so the ice-man never visited us.

Jackie and his friend Davy Kendrick and I would hide in the bushes and wait for the iceman to have his back turned and we would steal as many small chunks of ice that we could carry–in our shirts and pants–a real cool treat on blazing hot days. I had an old, two-wheeler bike that a friend of Dad's gave me that his daughter had outgrown and when something needed to be fixed on it, I would ride down to Jackie and he would spend hours fixing it for me. Summer afternoons were often interrupted by a visit from Aunt Nora! Aunt Nora was our Great Aunt because she was already Dad's aunt and Aunt Dot's aunt! She lived with her only child, Freddy, and his wife, Dot, whom everybody called *Crem* because her maiden name was Cremmins.

Aunt Nora loved kids! And especially she loved each one of us! She always had a candy bar in her hand bag for each of us! She never had much money, but she always had something in her bag for the kids! She hated Crem. Ma and Aunt Dot said Aunt Nora was jealous of Crem! When Aunt Dot looked out the sun-room window and saw Aunt Nora coming she would throw her head back and wail, "Holy God! It's Aunt Nora!" Aunt Nora was extremely hard of hearing. She yelled when she talked and we had to yell back at her and she'd bend over toward us and say, "Whaaat?" But when Aunt Nora got to the back door Aunt Dot was all smiles and greeted her as nice as you please, "Oh, Hi! Aunt Nora!" Aunt Nora helped Ma and Aunt Dot with their ironing and other household chores and worked at the Stoneham Laundry as well.

I really enjoyed those summer afternoons at Aunt Dot's when Jackie was around and there were things to do. Until one afternoon when I rode my bike down by myself and wandered into the cellar through the open bulk head door looking for Jackie. I saw a dirty faced mechanic guy who must have been helping Uncle Jack that day. He was standing in the coal bin, holding his big penis in his hands and staring out the cellar window at Bette Jean and her friend, Mary Lou who were dressed in shorts, doing cartwheels on the lawn. I was frozen to the spot, fidgeting my fingers together. "Just coolin' off," he said as he put his penis back in his pants and came over to me grinning as though I hadn't seen anything and he pulled me in front of him and touched me. I was scared but I liked how it felt when he touched me and how he talked softly to me, but I was still filled with fright at the same time, so I pulled away from him and ran outside to where Bette Jean and Mary Lou were. My Dad happened to come by a few minutes later and I told him that I didn't feel good and wanted to ride home with him. I left my bike there and Aunt Dot's house felt different to me after that. Whenever I was down there and glanced at that bulk head door, I would shiver inside, thinking that the man with the soft voice and dirty, ugly grinning face was always in there lurking somewhere and watching... me!

Shock

It was in the early morning of September, 1946 and Peggy and I were getting ready for school. The front door bell rang and Ma went to answer it. Dad's supervisor, Mr. Burg, was there with the Electric Company's Safety Inspector. Mr. Burg said that Dad had a serious accident. They sat down on the sofa in the living room. Ma sat down, too and Peggy and I sat beside Ma. There had been a power outage in Malden and Dad had been working under ground all night splicing and restoring cables. "The accident happened around 3:15 a.m." Mr. Burg said. "The doctors saved his eyesight but he had second degree burns on his face and third degree burns on his left arm. Fortunately, he had his safety gloves on and his hands were protected."

I was scared and moved close to Ma. She was silent but I knew she was scared, too. Mr. Burg was very kind. He spoke softly and directly to Ma. "Harry cut into a live cable," he said. Ma questioned that right away. "But he is always so cautious." "Yes," Mr. Burg said, "His cautious methods prevented him from being even more seriously injured—his boots, safety goggles and gloves. Many of the men don't always wear their safety equipment and sometimes incur even more dangerous injuries." He said that Dad was at the Widden Memorial Hospital in Everett.

Ma made up a quick cereal breakfast and sent Peggy and I off to school. Later Uncle Jack and Aunt Dot drove her to see Dad in the hospital. She told us that Dad's face was all black and swollen. Dad stayed in the hospital for two weeks and when he came home he was extremely nervous—and very unlike him, impatient with us. Ma told us that we must remember that Dad had been through a horribly frightening accident and his nerves were affected. I was worried about him all that time during his recovery. Ma too worried a lot after that.

Dad got better and went back to work in six weeks. He had a frightening looking scar on his left arm and on the inside of his elbow the skin was all white and wrinkled. He never wore short sleeve shirts after the accident. Other than that, he was okay!

There was a lot of talk about Dad's accident between Ma and Dad. Over and over, again and again, they talked about whose fault it was. Was the cable marked improperly or not at all? Dad was always so cautious. Why did he cut into a live cable? It was so unlike him. Safety first. That's what Dad believed. He was on the Safety First Committee. He even wrote a column for the company paper on safety. Dad was proud of his work on the committee, so it was hard for Ma to accept the accident as Dad's fault. And although he continued to believe that the cable was not marked, Dad was good friends with all of the men he worked with and no doubt wanted to keep the status quo in that. I never knew him to fight with his co-workers about anything–not any more than he would fight with his neighbors. He simply wasn't a fighter. Not even when he was right and someone else was wrong–even like in this issue, when he had to suffer the consequences. Ma was furious with him because of his unwillingness to stand up for himself.

Years earlier, when Dad was being promoted to First Class Cable Splicer, he didn't want the promotion. He kept declining it, until Mr. Burg came to the house, talked to Ma and encouraged her to talk Dad into accepting the promotion because not only did it mean a significantly higher salary for him and the family, but also that Dad belonged to the Union, had seniority and needed to take the promotion before others could move ahead. For some reason, maybe because he didn't want the added responsibility, Dad continued to reject the promotion. Ma kept on nagging him about it until he finally relented and took it. Ma continued to be angry with Dad for not taking it when it was first offered.

In its final assessment, the Company argued that the cable was marked and Dad likely had been overtired because he had worked all night and he must have accidentally cut into it. As a consequence, he lost his status as a First Class cable splicer. After that, because he lost his First Class status and the financial benefits that entailed, Ma lost whatever respect she had for Dad. He gave in to the pressure. He even said later that perhaps the cable was marked and maybe he did overlook it. He had, after all, worked all night.

Ma went silent. Cold. Distant. She had been all of that anyway, but now she had an excuse. Now she could say it was all Dad's fault. She was cold, distant and unloving. She could not stomach the fact that he would not fight for himself. They slept in twin beds anyway. Now they just rolled away from each other. Dad faced the far window. Ma turned and slept facing the door.

I would sometimes crawl into bed with Dad. He was snug and warm. I never got into bed with Ma.

The accident had established a clear and painful distance between them. Anytime Ma wanted to hurt Dad she'd make a reference to the accident. He knew and she knew. It was shameful. Ma made Dad cower. He never stood up to her. He would walk away. In time, all it took was a glance from Ma to do it.

Eventually, Dad had another accident on the job–a smaller one, yes, but larger in its consequences because he lost his job as a second class cable splicer altogether and was given instead a janitors job. Ma was wild about it, because Dad had to settle for a lessor salary. Again, he just took it. From that point on, Ma treated him like he was a boarder in his own house. I felt the coldness. I felt the distance. I stayed quiet. and still.

Peggy

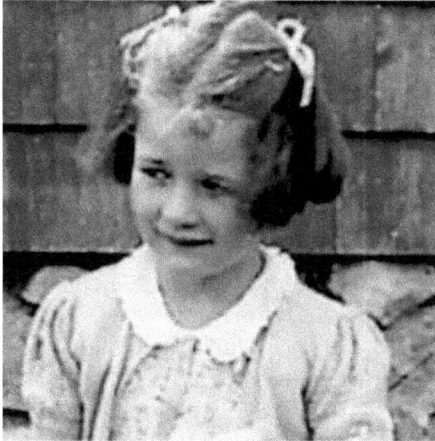

Grammar school

I was in first grade when Peggy was in fourth. Connie Elliott was a year older than Peggy and Tommy Elliott was a year older than me. We walked to school together during that first school year, because we had to cross Main Street and I wasn't allowed to cross that busy street alone at only six years old. Peggy would look back over her shoulder toward me, but I never knew whether she was making sure I was staying far enough away from her, or hoping that I was gone.

Ann Murphy had blond braids with her hair parted straight down the middle. She was older than me and stopped me on Pomworth Street and said I was *cross-eyed*. That was when I became aware of my eyes turning in. Ma said my eyes would turn in when I was tired. She and I took the street car to Malden where we went into an old brick building and took the elevator to the third floor where Dr. Haire, the eye doctor, examined my eyes. A year later, Dr. Haire operated on my eyes at Melrose Hospital. I remember the bed with rails and white bandages. I stayed quiet, but wasn't there long–only two days. After that my eyes were not crossed anymore.

I have flashes of sometimes liking Peggy–wanting to play with her–wanting to join in with her. There were occasional times when she was playful and carefree, not worried and angry. I saw her then and wanted to be with her. Peggy was athletic–good in sports and could play baseball with the big kids, like Beadie Viera, Allie Duff, Jimmy Duff and Connie Elliott. Peggy was good at whatever she did. She was smart in school and could and would do anything she wanted to do. Her friends seemed to like her for that sort of independence. And every once and a while she was actually nice to me. One of those times was on my birthdays. I thought at those times there was a possibility that *maybe* she did like me a little. I thought *maybe* we could be friends. But those times were short lived. As soon as I got lightened up and hopeful, she pulled the shade down. She turned stone cold, glared at me and turned me stone cold, too. I was sad and disappointed because Ma was like that too. I got hopeful around Ma sometimes–just like with Peggy. Ma would seem to get light and a brightness would shine in her and I'd get happy and begin to move toward that light, but when she caught a glimpse of me coming near her, a darkness would come over her and a coldness would engulf her. Then I would turn all cold and afraid and would stop just shy of her, like I would stop just shy of Peggy. I felt that hollowed-out-ness thing. That caved-in-ness. A kind of alone-ness that ate my insides out. It would work its way from my insides out, so that I couldn't let anything in. I felt poisoned, so much so that vomit would come up and stick in my throat so that nothing could fit in my mouth because my throat was shut tight to keep the vomit from exploding out of me.

All that horrid aloneness. That horridness of being pushed away.

"GET OUT OF HERE!" "GET AWAY FROM ME!" "STOP IT" "GO AWAY!" "GET OUT!" "DON'T COME NEAR ME!" And the door slammed in my face again and again. When Ma was dressing in her bedroom and I saw the half open door, if I moved toward the door Ma would scream, "GET OUT OF HERE!" And I would pull away from the door feeling that I'd done some awful thing.

I sought refuge in Dad's company. Dad said, "You stick with me Stevie." And I would do just that. We stuck together in his garden and in his Dark Room where he developed and enlarged the pictures he took. He'd speak about how to deal with Peggy. "Give it to her!" "Just give it to her," Dad would say when Peggy wanted what I had. "Just give it to her! And you come with me." And I did. I gave it to her and went with Dad, weakening and feeling even smaller than I was, leaving Peggy's anger just as strong as it was. Walking away made me sad and even being with Dad at those times made me feel lonely. I wanted to be friends with Peggy. I wanted her to show me how to play baseball. I wanted her to show me how to do the things she knew how to do. There was a pain in my stomach that would not go away. In bed at night I would pull my knees up under me and press them against my stomach to squeeze away the hurt. It stayed–a bleeding, aching hurt that never went away. A gaping hole that never got filled in. Even today, a knife cuts through my stomach when I think of those feelings–when I think of wanting to be friends with her and how afraid I was of opening up all that pain–reawakening all that vulnerability. Afraid I'd have to *give* it to her. Just *give* it to her. Afraid she would annihilate me. Kill me. Cut me into pieces. Shred me. Slice me into thin, raw slices until I bled to death. NO! NO! NO! I don't want her near me! Keep her away from me! Not now! Not ever! KEEP HER AWAY!

Ma's way of talking about Peggy Ann was so different from her way of talking about me, which was favorable. Favorable meant "more like her." Unfavorable meant " more like Dad." Ma's stories about Peggy are more real in my memory than Peggy herself. As early as I can remember, Ma told stories of how Peggy was as a baby and as a toddler. She said Peggy was a serious baby, hardly ever smiled–said she had a mean deposition even when she was a toddler. "She was born that way," Ma said. She scratched the face of a girl named Mary Ann who came to visit. Mary Ann was Peggy's age and when she sat in Peggy's rocking chair, Peggy went over and scratched her face so that it bled. Ma was shocked and embarrassed! She said whenever she'd hear a child crying outside she figured that Peggy had probably done something to hurt the child. She would pull off their hair ribbons, hit them, twist their arms or otherwise hurt them. She loved to give Indian burns to kids she didn't like. Ma said she couldn't understand Peggy's behavior and she said Mrs. Elliott couldn't understand Peggy either. Ma figured Peggy must be like "the Duffys" because no one on her side of the family had a mean streak like that.

Ma didn't know much about kids or babies. She was thirty when Peggy was born and Dad was thirty-six. She had worked in Boston for thirteen years before she married Dad. She was very proud of herself, her job, her looks and her clothes. The photos of her from that time show her as attractive, fashionable, stiff, cold and distant. "Miss Lee. Dorothy Margaret Lee."

Men were readily attracted to her wiles, but as soon as she sensed their capitulation, she would quickly and easily deflect their advances, as they were no match to the incomparable loving memories of her red-headed Joe, so thoroughly embedded and alive in her thoughts and day dreams.

Ma said that Peggy's sallow complexion and olive coloring was probably caused by poor blood–so unlike her own high color. Ma was so proud of her nice complexion and good looks. She held her head high, showing no trace of shame or any sort of inadequacy. She said that I had her light complexion, but not her high color. When we were out shopping Ma would point out other people's daughters who weren't as pretty as their mothers. Ma was sorry that none of us children had Dad's violet-blue eyes and coal-black hair. Ma was proud of Dad's good looks as she was proud of her own. Peggy looked more like Dad, but Ma was oblivious to that natural beauty. She chose to see her flaws–her inadequacies–like the skin blemishes of adolescence. Ma never had a blemish. She seemed to look at it as a character deficiency. So it wouldn't reflect on her, she saw to it that Peggy went to a dermatologist. "Must be something wrong with her blood," she would say repeatedly. To be perfectly honest, I didn't think Peggy was that pretty either, maybe because she carried so much anger and harbored such a mean disposition.

Ma constantly made comments how Peggy was making her front teeth protrude by sucking her thumb so much, so she made sure Peggy saw an Orthodontist for braces. Ma often told Peggy that she needed to get her blood checked, because she might be anemic. Ma prided herself for having an even temperament. She would compare Peggy's sour disposition to her own pleasant disposition. She would lapse into reverie as she told us how at the office, everyone liked "Miss Lee" and how Salesmen would ask specifically to speak with Miss Lee because of her pleasant manner and even temperament. Ma told endless stories of "Miss Lee." She told us about her pretty clothes, her hats and gloves and *I. Miller* shoes, her Raccoon coats–two of them, no less! Ma described in detail outfits that were especially striking. She said she was talked about as the best dressed girl in West Lynn. And the most religious! (How she became privy to that information I have no idea.) Ma was a Daily Communicant at church. She loved to talk about her devotion to The Sacred Heart of Jesus and the Souls in Purgatory. On her lunch hour she would leave the office and rush over to St. James Church for Holy Hour. All in all, in Ma's eyes, she was just about perfect. She was so, so proud when she was chosen to be "Prefect" of Our Lady's Sodality!

Ma said Peggy was more like Dad and Aunt Dot's mother, Ma Duffy cranky, crabby and bossy. Ma denied any wrong doing on her part in dealing with Peggy as a totally unjust, unthinkable accusation. "Why no child ever wanted more than Peggy!" she'd say. But Peggy continued to crash into Ma's day dreams demanding her attention. She needed Ma's affection. But Ma refused to detach herself from her precious memories and pay attention to her baby girl. So Peggy reamed Ma every chance she got with her awful behavior. They screamed at each other.

I caught on early–didn't get Ma's attention or affection either, but my way of responding was different. I watched Peggy and Ma from a distance and I was afraid of both of them, so deciding to be quiet was the best way–stay away, shut my mouth and keep it shut.

I resisted Ma's aloofness by not eating! But because I stayed quiet, Ma found me easier than Peggy. Ma said favorable things about me. She said I took after her side of the family–that my light skin was like hers and burned easily in the summer. She would say that I had inherited her even disposition and was easy to get along with. She never knew that was because of my own choice to never cause any trouble. I saw Ma and Peggy at the center of our family stage, locked in rage and screaming at each other and stayed as far away from the tumultuous drama that I could–as far away as I could possibly go.

None of us, not Peggy, not Paul and not me, ever shined as brightly as Ma telling stories of her school days–how she was Sister Christina's pet. She was best at just about everything! Playing the Organ. Leading the Rosary. Memorizing poems. Reciting lessons in class. Ma was just about perfect! At school. At work. And lest we forgot, "the best looking too!"

Peggy was smart in school–an *all A* student in the fourth grade, even though she hated St. Pat's school and the nuns. The Sisters of Providence who taught at St. Pat's were harsh and critical. They were a lot like Ma, but Ma had only good things to say about them. I don't know of any one of the nuns who was popular or well liked by the kids! I didn't like most of them and Peggy disliked them all. I did half like Sister Mary Gonzaga, but even at that I saw through her and realized she gave special attention to kids who got sick. Peggy just wanted to get out of that school after eighth grade. The eighth grade teacher, Sister Dorothy Marie, accused Peggy of looking out the window in the direction of the Public High and told her she'd be there soon enough and to stop looking out the window! Peggy continued to look out the window until the day she left and finally got to High School. As soon as she stepped through the front door of Stoneham High School she began to sparkle! At Stoneham High she was not only bright and popular, but she loved her teachers and she had lots of friends! Even Ma began to take notice of the "Cinderella" like transformation.

She began to radiate and flashed a brand new smile. She used makeup to bring out her gray eyes clearer. She brought high color to her cheeks with just the right amount of make-up and red lipstick to outline her smile, revealing her small, but evenly aligned white teeth. She wore her hair in a poodle cut. She was pert and sassy– popular with her teachers, her classmates and especially the boys!

To make sure she didn't ever get to feel too good about herself, Ma brought out more and more of her own stories of her youth, beauty and boyfriends and showed Peggy how she should be in the world, all the while criticizing her for being the way she was! It was hard for Peggy to keep the spotlight on herself for long at home, because Ma would call her *Miss Scarlett O'Hara* and tell her that she would burn in hell for flirting with the boys.

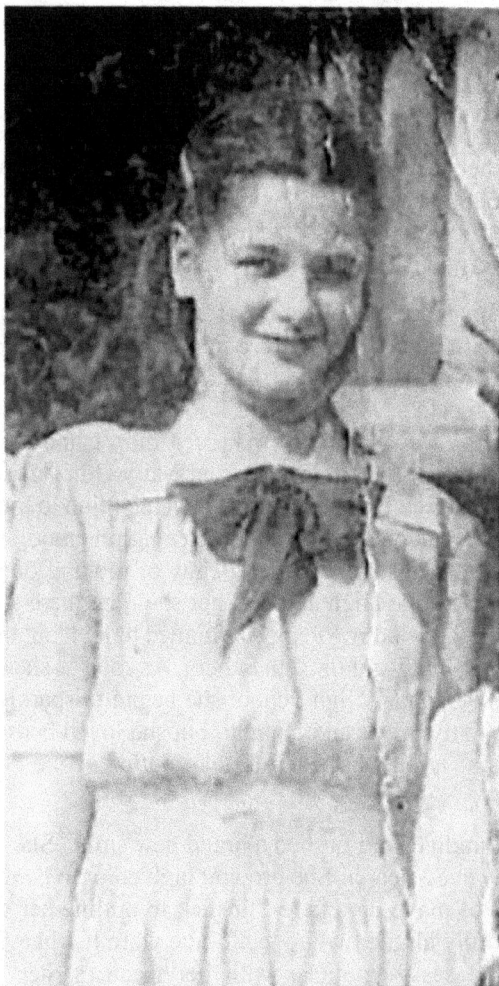

Peggy, Jr. High School

I myself was conflicted about Peggy. The meanness and cranky disposition was still there at home. Ma said she was a house devil and a street angel. That was Ma's surface answer as to what made Peggy, tick.

Ma continued to stay caught up in her memories. Her real world never even near to matching the cinema-scope memories she had created of her life before Dad. She never learned how to comfortably hold a baby in her arms and give of herself. She never learned to fill a baby's insatiable hunger to feel love. The baby was but a chore to get done according to the rules of Dr. Spock and Mrs. Elliott. She did her duty and she did it faithfully in the *right* way. She took her responsibilities seriously.

Peggy's anger reflected much of what was wrong in our household.

Her anger gave expression to the unspoken pain we all felt–the secrets, the broken hearts and the lies. She reflected the pent up frustrations, the darkness of spirit. She acted out and the rest of us pointed and said," She's mean! She's selfish! She's a dog in the manger!" But today, the professional care givers might say she was the obvious victim of family dysfunction caused by adult children of alcoholic grand-parents. Being the oldest, she was psychologically together enough to protest her chains and lash out in defiance and anger.

I was perplexed by Peggy's behavior toward me. She would pose in front of me, hand on hip, jutting her chin and hips out and fluffing her hair, as though I was a mirror. She would stick her face in mine with a sly look saying in a sing songy voice, "Mirror, mirror on the wall, who is the fairest of them all?" insisting that I notice how pretty she was, how strong, how athletic. She would mimic swim strokes, saying:" Wouldn't you just love to be able to swim like me? I love to feel the water in my face and swim through the waves!" I would be anchored in my wheelchair in the breezeway–confined, sweating in the summer heat, unable to do or be anywhere else just then, and I was bewildered by her attitude that seemed to be intentionally hurtful. I was more struck by her behavior than I was by my deprivation. I would watch her and Ma from a safe distance. Polio rescued me and in that one big way; I was out of the running. I didn't have to compete! I didn't relate to any of it, but somehow I watched. I wondered. I tried to make sense out of it all. I couldn't understand what sense it made for girls to grow up and do the whole thing all over again. I mean, to get married and have more babies and bring them up so they'd get married and have even more babies. I remember listening to Ma and watching Peggy–thinking how out of kilter it was. None of it made sense and it threatened me in ways I could not grasp. Sometimes when my guard was down even polio couldn't exclude me. I was afraid Peggy would annihilate me–kill me– take my breath away. Snuff the life out of me! Other times I felt compassion for Peggy. I saw her vulnerability through her transparent skin. The way her veins popped up through her temples and on the back of her hands.

When I looked toward her for any sort of help, most of the time I would get, "get away from me. I can't help you." She had all she could do to *survive*! Stoneham High School was the main stage for her–topped off with the lead role in the Senior Play, "Father of the Bride" and ending with getting voted Prettiest Girl in the Senior Class, then finally graduating with honors and nothing would or could ever take the place of all that success and celebrity and her past, like Ma's, became her future, while Polio provided a totally other arena for me to play out my own existential estrangement.

Meals

Ma prided herself on being well organized. As strictly as she practiced her religion, she did her sacred tasks–cleaning the house, doing the laundry, grocery shopping and cooking. Every Monday morning she washed the clothes in the deep set tub of the kitchen sink. She scrubbed each piece on the scrub-board then wrung them out by hand and hung them on the clothesline in the back yard next to Dad's flower garden. Dad said we didn't need a washing machine because the McAuliffe's didn't have one. Ma resented that Dad decided whether or not to purchase things she needed based on what the McAuliffe's had or didn't have. It further disturbed her because both Mrs. Elliott and Mrs. Gusterferro had a washer and a dryer.

In winter the clothes would sometimes freeze on the line and become all stiff like rigor-mortis. Ma would soften them limp by spreading them on clothes racks in the kitchen and laying them over the radiators in the other rooms. One extremely cold winter day Dad's union-suit flew off the line and landed in the Elliott's back yard, fifty feet away from our house. It lay there swollen, stiff and frozen until Mrs. Elliott directed four-year-old Tommy to pull it back over to our house. We were all obliviously eating supper when we heard a wailing sound coming from outside. Peggy's seat was closest to the door so Ma told her to go see what it was. Peggy looked out the door and came back into the kitchen unsuccessfully suppressing a giggle. That inspired the rest of us to go to the door. It was a sight to behold–a frozen union-suit tumbling in the wind over the snow, with a hysterical "never give up" Tommy hanging on to one of the frozen legs for dear life.

Dad ran out and pried Tommy off the union-suit and we all had a good laugh... except for Tommy who stood there bawling, afraid that his Mommy would be mad because he didn't do the job like his Mommy told him to.

Ma ironed on Tuesday and baked on Wednesday. She took great pride in her cooking and deservedly so, making sure all of her meals were well balanced. She planned her weekly menu carefully–a roast on Sunday heated over for Monday night's supper. Tuesday was chops or chicken and Wednesday could be creamed-chip-beef and mashed potatoes or baked macaroni and stewed tomatoes. Thursday was a meat loaf or beef stew. In those days being Catholic meant fish on Fridays and on Saturdays we had beans and franks! When we didn't have a roast on Sunday we had home made chicken soup or ham. Ma loved ham and lots of times we had a boiled dinner with a smoked shoulder, cabbage and boiled potatoes, with spare ribs on the side! Jello or tapioca pudding were easy deserts when Ma didn't have time to bake a pie. And she had her special pies! *Lemon meringue* was her favorite and mine! Dad loved blueberry pie made from the preserved berries he had picked the summer before.

Meals were always perfectly arranged by Ma. We had a drop leaf table in the kitchen. It was painted green and the wooden chairs were green to match. The table was in front of the window that looked out at the Elliott's house. At suppertime, we had to pull the table out and extend the two leaves. I sat near the window and my chair was up against the radiator. I felt that I had the best seat because the heater warmed my back in winter and I had the coolness of the open window in the summer. Just outside the window there was a bridal wreath bush that every June was covered with white blossoms. Dad sat to my left at the head of the table and Ma straight across and Paul's high chair was at the corner between Ma and Dad and Peggy sat at the end of the table opposite Dad with her back to the hallway leading outside. Meal time was a strain on me because I had difficulty swallowing, so I would spend most of the time moving the food around on my plate, trying to make it look like I was eating more than I was. Ma would comment on my pretend eating and accuse me of spoiling my meals by eating candy–even when I hadn't. She made me anxious the way she would watch me and keep telling me I had to eat. All that watching made me uncomfortable.

5-10 Years

McKenna's General Store was on the corner of Main Street and Montvale Ave and on Saturdays Ma would take me by the hand and walk up there for groceries. In winter she would bundle me up in a warm afghan and pull me behind her on a sled. Then we would go beyond McKenna's all the way to Stoneham Square to McDonough's Market, because World War II had imposed certain restrictions on citizens and Ma had ration cards for butter, sugar and meat and McDonough's market carried all three items. While in the square, we would go into Woolworth's Five and Ten Cent store and the Middlesex Drug Store and if we had time we would go into to Helen Fitzpatrick's Vogue (Notions) Shop to say hello to Jackie and Bette's Aunt Katherine, who worked there and we all called her Aunt Katherine too.

During those five through ten years, Ma relived her life-time memories to me over and over–*her* childhood–*her* favorite dress–*her* favorite teacher–*her* favorite book–*her* favorite friend... on and on. When we were together, Ma seemed like a blind lady who couldn't see me. She was so lost in her thoughts and memories I might as well not even have been there, but on the other hand, she had no one else there to listen.

Later on, when Polio wouldn't allow me to loco-mote. Ma had a captive audience and began to share the darker side of her reality as a little girl. She told me that Nana was a drunk–that her earliest memories were of her mother flat on the floor dead drunk. When that would happen, which was frequently, Alice, would become hysterical with fright and Holidays became nightmares of barren drunkenness. Grampa faded helplessly into the background and Ma was left all alone to deal with it. I became her lone invisible listener–quiet, unseen, and unheard.

When I was nine I had a love affair with Peggy's pale-blue two-wheeled bike, which she no longer used. The tires were thin but strong and it was just the right size for me. In the summer evenings after supper, I would go on what I liked to call, "My personal journey of left turns." Dad would be up on the porch reading the Boston Globe, smoking his pipe and rocking in his rocking chair with his stocking feet propped up on the screened-in window sill. I would take the bike out of the garage, look up at Dad's toes, hop on and peddle a hundred yards up Cottage Street toward William Street.

What inspired me most, was the great sense of mastery I had on that bike! It was fast and I felt strong–un-stoppable and flushed with excitement as I whizzed by Judy Burke's house, took a left onto William Street, sailed down the hill and turned left on West Street, sailing by all the nice houses with the finely manicured lawns that lined both sides of the street and then turned left again onto Lindenwood Rd. up the hill to the corner of Cottage St. by the Monarch's house, making the fourth left, back onto Cottage, flying downhill past the Bauer's house and peddling hard again until I stopped right in front of Dad's toes and curling pipe smoke again. I would keep taking the same route again and again, all the time humming to myself Gene Autry's famous song, *"Over and Over and over and over again"* until the streetlights came on and Dad called down to me, "Come on in now Stevie. Put the bike away. It's getting too dark for you to be out there. Come on in now."

I loved those warm summer evenings!

I started off to the first grade with the excitement of new clothes, new stuff to learn, new kids to meet–all who seemed more savvy and life aware than me. Some of the neighborhood kids went to the Emerson School and some to the North School where Jackie and Bette Flynn went. The new Robin Hood School was built the year I got Polio and Jackie transferred there when he was twelve.

So to make sure her Faith was passed on to her children, Ma would entertain no other notion than Catholic Schools for me and Peggy.

I remember my first day in First Grade when Sister Rose Eleanor closed the classroom door on Jean McCarthy's finger. Jean stood there with her bloody red socks matching the red bow in her hair with Sister beside her stemming the blood flow and giving her hugs of consolation. I didn't feel consoled in that musty old classroom. I felt lonely–especially later on in that school year, I was stunned and ashamed when Sister Rose Eleanor gave me a smack across my head for gazing out the window.

And I felt shamed and bewildered in the second grade when Sister Gertrude Irene called Peggy into the classroom after school to show her my messy desk. She asked Peggy to help me straighten it out. The kids liked Sister Gertrude Irene. I didn't. And I positively hated Sister Marie Veronica! She was my third grade teacher. Her face was stern and pock marked from smallpox. I made a mistake every single time I got up to read and she would make me go to the end of the line. I would make repetitive mistakes at the blackboard in arithmetic and regularly was told to sit down. My self esteem had no chance at all in her classroom. I shriveled before her constant unnerving glare of criticism and disapproval.

Sister Gertrude Delores was the terror of Fourth Grade. The boys were terrified of her reputation for slamming their heads into the blackboard during arithmetic class. She did it routinely. Just as routinely as she stepped into the supply closet with her back to the class while she opened a thermos and drank its contents at ten o'clock every morning. She held a clicker when we were doing reading exercises and clicked it instead of saying "next". She would click on Eleanor Meuse as soon as Eleanor made a mistake, which was almost immediately every time. But somehow I managed to hold my own in that Fourth Grade.

The first few days of Fifth Grade held out the hope that I might actually like school that year for a change. Sister Mary Gonzaga smiled right at me from the start. She liked me! She actually liked me! I might even go so far as to say, I was her pet. Sister would call on me to lead the Rosary. "*Barbara Lee!*" she would call out. "Come lead the Rosary." In the school play my name was *Charity* and the kids teased me about the name, until Sister Gertrude confided to me that charity meant *love* and after that the kid's jealousy didn't bother me one single bit.

She wrote her name on the blackboard and made sure we knew how to spell G-o-n-z-a-g-a! Sister Mary Gonzaga! She said the number "5" was like a man running with his hat on! And she also said to color round and round and round in circles so the lines wouldn't show.

It was easy to go to the blackboard in Sister Mary Gonzaga's classroom and it was easy to stand up and recite in her room too. All of that made the Fifth Grade a pleasant place to be.

Totsie Johnson got hit by a truck that year and Laura Jackson had Rheumatic Fever. Sister Mary Gonzaga was very concerned and gave each of them lots of attention when they came back to school. Jimmy Keagan (my boyfriend since the fourth grade) moved away to Malden that year. Jimmy lived on Collincote Street across the street from Aunt Nora. We sat side by side on the curb in front of Aunt Nora's house one afternoon eating ice cream cones. I remember feeling lonesome and very sad when his family moved and the class said Good Bye to him.

After fifth grade, during the summer, I got Polio and never went back to St. Pat's as a student again.

There were some bright moments in those early years, but most of them were away from home. When I turned ten, I took piano lessons with Kathy English who lived in a large Victorian house on Maple Street. I wasn't very good at playing the piano and when I played the wrong keys Kathy would put her head back and say, "Oh, my aching back!" I liked walking to Kathy's house after school in the Fall because there were very old, trees on Maple Street and the leaves covered the sidewalk and were wonderful to walk through. The leaves flew in the air and crackled and crunched under my feet. A wooden porch wrapped all around the front of Kathy's house and there were two Baby Grand pianos in her spacious front room. Kathy was planning to be married and one afternoon she showed me the material for her wedding dress. It was in the lower drawer of the buffet in the dining room. Everything about Kathy and her house was like a dream.

On Saturday mornings Kathy had a club for her piano students and she invited me to come. She told me to come to the back door at nine a.m. Although both Peggy and Bette Jean took piano from Kathy, I don't think they ever went to her club. One Saturday I went there by myself. I got there at nine o'clock as Kathy said and I went to the back door. I stood at the foot of the steps and didn't know what to do. Kathy had said, "Come to the back door." That was all she said, so with no other instructions to be guided by, I did just that–stood there. Finally Kathy's mother, Mrs. English, happened to come out and asked me if I needed help. I said, "No." And I continued to stand there feeling extremely embarrassed and awkward. Finally, after what seemed a very long time, Kathy came out of another door around the back of the house and said, It's eleven o'clock. The class is all over." "How long have you been here? I felt ashamed and embarrassed. I felt *so* stupid!

Kathy got married that summer. The same summer I caught Polio. She came to see me in the hospital and told me all about her wedding. She brought brownies she had baked. I liked Kathy, a lot!

Around that same time I found a new friend, Seven-year-old Estelle. Estelle was a little ragamuffin girl. Her mother owned the Friendly Variety Store on Main Street next to the railroad tracks. She had really pretty hair– very long, light brown and curly, almost gold! Her hair never looked combed– it was just there–all over her head and framing her soft pretty face. Her dresses, socks and shoes were like her hair–rumpled, messy and dirty. I liked Estelle a lot! She was full of energy and fun and easy to be with. She smiled all the time and liked to play with me. She was always dancing and prancing, wasn't shy at all and not aware that when she lifted her leg over the baton everyone could see her dirty underpants. She was rarely seen not twirling her baton and told everyone she met that she was going to be a majorette when she got bigger. Ma didn't like her. Her mother only owned the store for a little while. Then Charlie bought the Variety Store and Estelle never came back.

Island Falls

It was in August of 1949. I had just turned ten. We Duffys–Harry, Dorothy, Peggy, little Paul and myself, and the Flynns–Uncle Jack, Aunt Dot (Dorothy) Bette Jean and Jackie went on vacation to Island Falls, Maine. It was after Nana and Grampa had died. Ma got some money from Grampa's Insurance, which enabled Dad to buy the only new car he ever owned–a 1949 gray Plymouth which he kept like new for thirteen years.

Flo McAuliffe and Marie owned Camp Theodore Roosevelt on Pleasant Lake, in northern Maine, about 165 miles south of New Brunswick, Canada. The camp consisted of a Main house, four cottages and two log cabins. There was also a large dining room where they served stacks of pancakes on Sunday Mornings. Flo had wanted Dad to come up for years.

I was excited all summer long waiting for Dad's vacation to hurry up and was especially glad that Jackie Flynn would be there too. Ma bought me a new outfit–a blue denim jacket with big pockets that came to my hips and had a hat to match. And I had plaid shorts. I felt wonderful in that outfit! Dad always took his vacation the last two weeks in August and Uncle Jack took his vacation then, too, so we could all go to Island Falls together. We started out early that Saturday morning, knowing that Uncle Jack was a slow starter and wouldn't get on the road with his 1939 Suburban much before noon. Dad wanted to arrive in camp as early as possible that night. It was about three hundred and fifty miles and he figured the trip would take about ten hours. Dad planned to stop in Bangor for a late lunch and groceries and the Camp was about a hundred miles from there.

Dad said Uncle Jack would catch up because he drove fast. Dad didn't like to drive as fast as Uncle Jack and he said there was no need to drive so fast if you got an early start. But Dad wasn't surprised when Uncle Jack caught up with us in Bangor. Uncle Jack yelled out the car window "I knew we'd catch up to ya." Dad didn't say anything back but he knew Uncle Jack must have really been speeding to catch up. Uncle Jack always acted like he thought he was smarter than Dad. I didn't think so. He was just louder and bragged a lot.

It was dark when we pulled into Camp and Flo and Marie and their kids, Johnny and Joanie came over to the cars to welcome us. Uncle Jack made a big deal right away about catching up. Flo didn't take notice. He was just so glad to have Dad there because they were such great pals. They loved to go fishing which they did day and night. Uncle Jack went along one day and got a terrible sunburn.

Aunt Dot, Uncle Jack, Bette Jean and Jackie had one big cottage. Ma, Peggy and two year old Paul had a cottage and Dad and I had one all to ourselves. We had the cottage on the knoll which was smaller than all the rest. It was the one Ma and Dad had stayed in when they went to Island Falls on their Honeymoon. Our cottage had an outhouse. The others had indoor toilets. There was no electricity and we used kerosene lamps when it got dark.

It was a great vacation because our cottages were just a short distance from the water's edge. All we had to do was walk out the door and into the lake! It was wonderful! The early morning sunshine sparkled on the water and made me squint my eyes in the brightness. The docks went straight out into the water and the row boats were tied up to each dock. Canoes were hanging from a rack nearby as well. For the good swimmers, there was a raft anchored about a hundred and fifty feet out from shore.

Jackie and I were in the water most of the day, every day. We loved the boats. Paul played at the water's edge and liked to throw small stones into the lake. Bette Jean and Peggy found a flat rock away from the cottages where they sunbathed each day. Bette Jean didn't like to get wet, but Peggy loved to dive off the flat rock and swim out to the Raft.

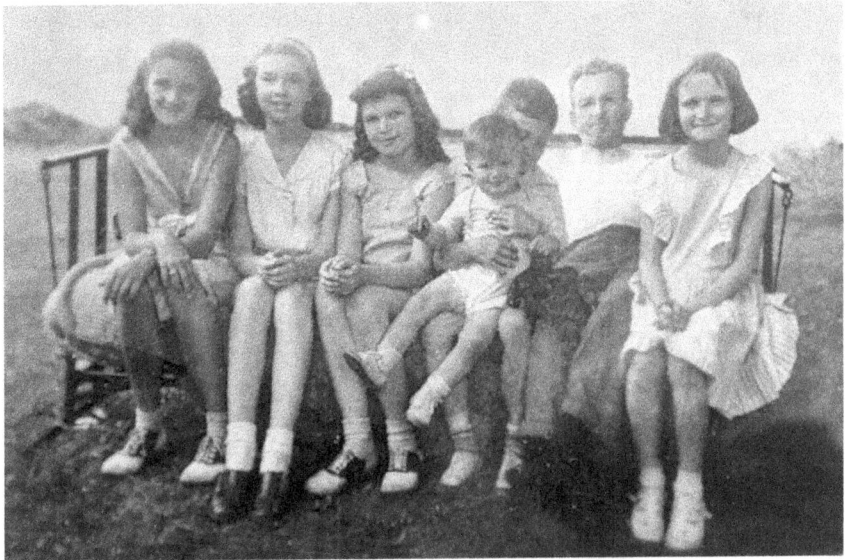

Peggy, Clair, Bette Jean, Paul, Jackie, Uncle Jack, Barbara

One day we all took a trip to New Brunswick Canada. It was so exciting to cross the border into another country. We had lunch in Canada. It was on that day that Ma and Uncle Jack had a fight. It was over Bette Jean. Ma said something about Bette Jean that made Uncle Jack mad. He yelled at Ma and told her never to say anything about Bette Jean again. Ma didn't like Uncle Jack anyway and was just as glad to have nothing more to do with him for the rest of the trip. Dad got nervous and was really mad at Ma for making the crack about Bette Jean in the first place.

Flo and Marie McAuliffe liked having us all there. In the evenings the adults would gather together at the main house and engage in lively political discussions, with the most contention between Marie and Uncle Jack. Ma and Marie were good friends. Marie resented the way Aunt Dot Flynn constantly made out how special Bette Jean was, as if she was better than the rest of us. Marie thought her kids were pretty special too. At their mother's prompting, they would show us their school papers that were covered with gold stars. She thought her daughter Joanie was just

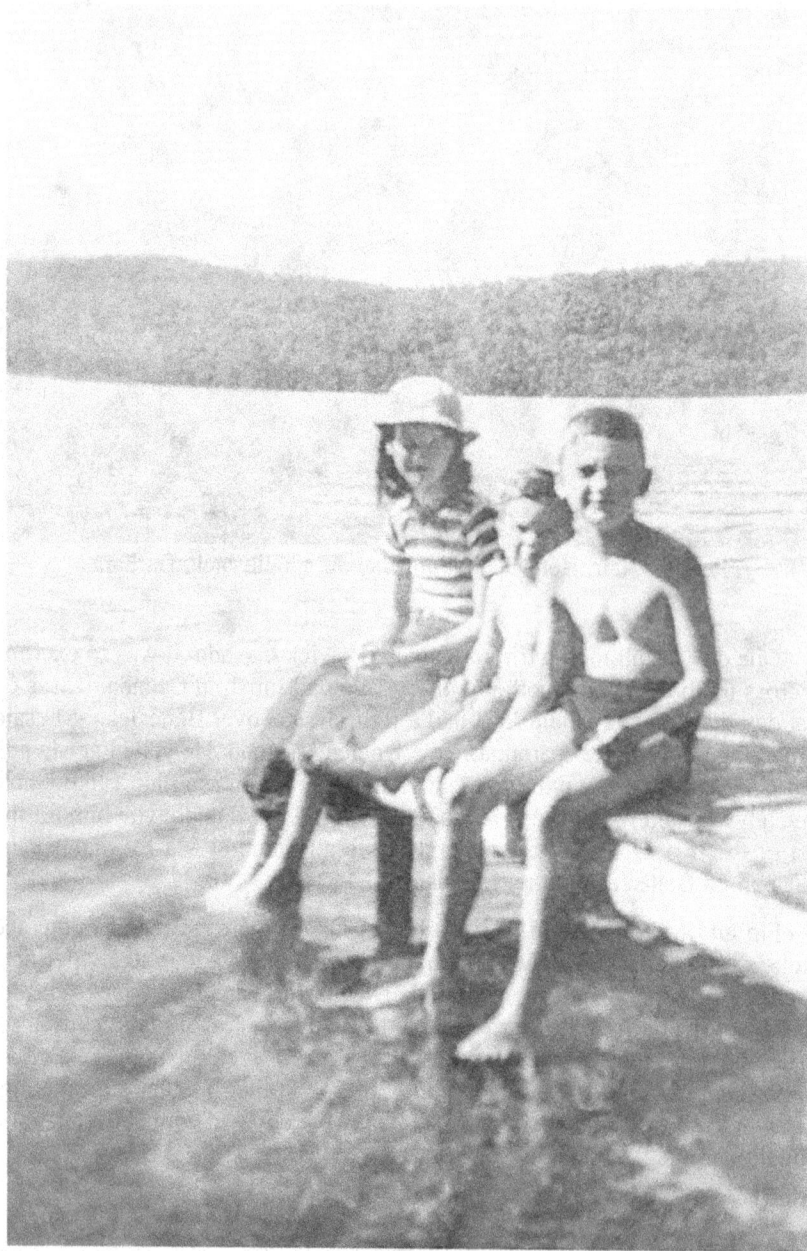

Barbara, Paul, Jackie

as pretty and smart as Bette Jean, which she was. Bette got all of her mother's attention and Jackie got little to none. Mostly, she left him alone to fend for himself, but she kept Bette Jean apart, unruffled and prettied up all of the time.

It was our best vacation ever, but in two weeks it was all over. When we came home, Dad promised that we would go back again next August.

The following July I got Polio and my biggest regret was that we never got to go back to Island Falls.

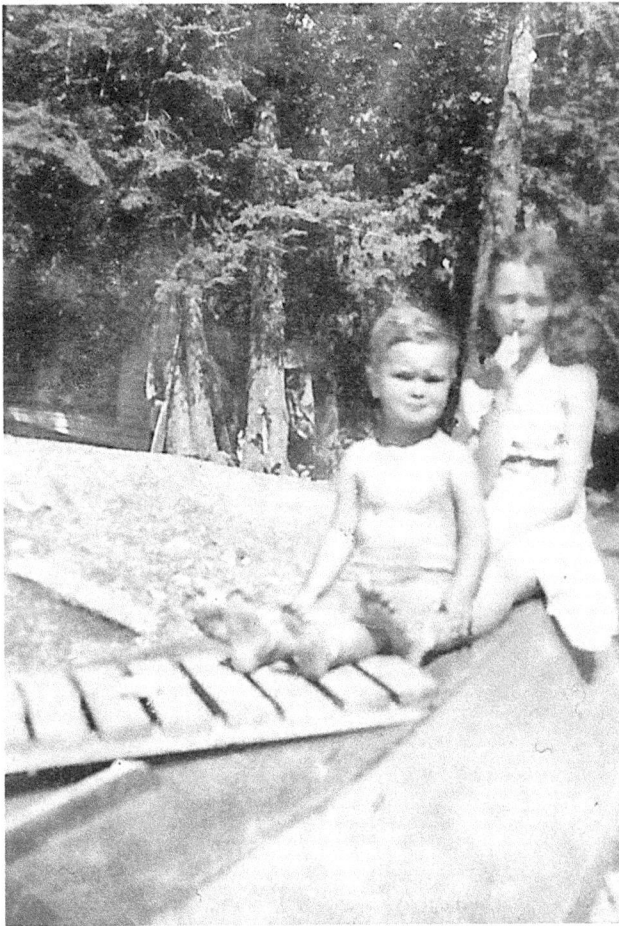

Paul & Barbara

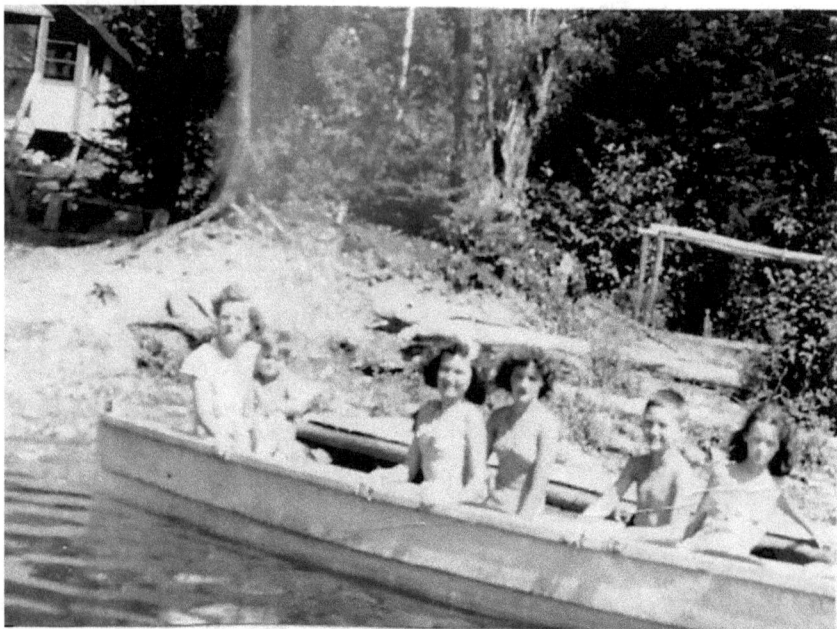

Ma, Paul, Bette Jean, Peggy, Jackie, Barbara

PART TWO

POLIO

I stood next to Ma as she did the supper dishes. It was summer. I asked her, "Ma, what's infantile paralysis?" I felt small standing there with one foot on top of the other. I don't remember what Ma said. I do remember that she answered me. She probably said it was an illness that crippled children.

It was the 4th of July and I was with Dad at the Common in Wakefield waiting for the fireworks. I felt tired, sat down on the ground and didn't run around as I usually did. Around that time I had an abscessed tooth and the dentist pulled it, leaving a huge hole in the back of my mouth. It was next to the last big tooth on the left bottom row of teeth. My tongue sought out the hole and probed it. That hole had a weirdness to it. At the Movies on Saturday afternoon I paid more attention to the hole than I paid to the movie. It had an unfamiliar taste.

It was an extremely hot day—a Friday. Aunt Dot called Ma. She said "Jack has the day off and we're going to Lynn Beach. Do you and Barbara want to come along?" Ma said that she had too much work to do but, "Barbara can go." Her response both surprised and pleased me, so I did go. It got really cool at the beach and felt like rain. I was chilled and walked around wrapped up in a towel. I stayed out of the water, which was unusual for me.

The following Sunday afternoon, Ma, Dad, Me Paul and Joey Gallella, an eight year old from up the street, went for a ride to Stage Fort Park in Gloucester, where we climbed the huge rocks that looked out to ward the open sea. We stayed all afternoon and on the way home we stopped for ice cream. At home in the kitchen, I told Ma I didn't feel good and she said I probably ate the ice cream too fast on such a hot day. I was sick during the night and stayed sick all the next day. Dr. Kliner came by on Tuesday and said I had a summer bug. He wasn't my regular Doctor and only came because our family doctor, Dr. Burke, was on vacation during July. Because it was a reoccurring problem with me, Ma always worried about me not eating, but this time she was more worried than usual. I was sick all day Wednesday and stayed on the sofa in the living room until I got up to go upstairs to the bathroom. I fell on the bottom step and was too weak to walk up the stairs. On Thursday I stayed in bed—in Dad's bed, not my own. Every time I took a sip of water, I choked. I was scared. Ma confided to her friend, Mrs. Gallella, that if she were an alarmist she'd say I had polio.

Dr. Kliner came again. This time he said I had to go to the hospital. Ma and Dad had a choice–Children's Hospital or another Boston hospital. I'd been to Children's as an infant, so they choose Children's again. Ma called Aunt Dot and Dad carried me from the bedroom to the cellar and into the garage, where he put me in the back seat with Aunt Dot. I sat on her lap, wrapped up in a blanket even though it was July 19th. We were all scared, so no one talked. Dad had trouble finding the hospital and drove into the driveway of the Angel Memorial Veterinary Hospital. We finally found the right place and some people came out with a stretcher and took me inside to a small examining room where I laid on a hard table for a long time. The doctors asked me questions and had me repeat "Peter Piper picked a peck of pickled peppers." They put a needle in my back to withdraw spinal fluid. After awhile the doctors decided that I must stay and Ma and Dad and Aunt Dot should go home. I felt very small. Then they put me on another stretcher and covered me with a sheet. Even my head because we were going into the elevator and what I had might be catching. I was taken upstairs to Isolation. They told me not to worry because Ma and Dad would come back tomorrow. All the people there were big and strong and knew what they were doing. All I had to do was lie there and be really quiet. I watched and watched–staying very still–didn't move even the tiniest muscle. It was a small dark room and only dim lights were on.

They told me then about the Iron Lung. "Like a big can," they said–"a very big, yellow can."

I felt infinitesimally tiny as I watched the huge yellow tank roll in through the door. It filled most of the room. The nurse opened the tank.

She pulled it apart and there was a bed inside. She demonstrated–laid down on it and said it was comfortable. I remained perfectly quiet as they picked me up and laid me down in the big yellow machine. They asked me how I was doing and I said OK. Before Each step, they told me what they were going to do. They said that they were going to slide me up a little so my head would stick out, while all the rest of me would be in the tank. That was scary. They went very slowly and after a few tries they got my head through the round opening in the top of the machine and then they slowly rolled the can so that it shut tight. They asked if I was still OK and I said yes. And they clamped it shut tight with big silver clamps. BOOMP! BOOMP! And then they turned it on WHOOOOOOOOSH!!! There was a huge big push inside and they said the machine would breathe for me. I didn't know what to do. How to breathe–in or out? So I asked them. "How do I breathe?" And the big machine swallowed up my words. My breath got all sucked away. The nurse stood by my head and told me to relax and just let the machine breathe for me.

I couldn't understand that and I tried to keep breathing–In and out. In and out. There was a sponge rubber tan cuff all around my neck. It puffed out and got sucked in–it puffed out and got sucked in–and then I knew–to breathe in when it puffed out and to breathe out when it got sucked in. It was confusing though and the more I thought about it the more mixed up I got. I tried to forget about it, but I kept watching the sponge rubber cuff as it puffed out and got sucked in–and after a while I learned to breathe in and out with the rubber cuff.

Soon the room grew light with daylight. I could see the yellowness of the big machine. My head rested on a pillow. They attached a mirror above my face and I could look into the mirror and see the door to my room behind me. Beyond the door was a hallway and a nurses' desk. Under the mirror and to my right on the yellow part of the machine there was a row of numbers. The numbers described the big machine. Later on I memorized all the numbers, but at first all I had to do was lie very still and let the machine do its work. The nurses wanted me to pee. They made a big deal about that. They kept the water running in the small sink and encouraged me to pee. It was hard to pee lying down and using a bedpan. When I finally did, everyone was very pleased. It was hard to drink anything. Because when I swallowed I choked. It was hard to know when to swallow. Like do I swallow when I breathe in, or when I breathe out? I followed the movement of the tan yellow cuff–do I swallow now? or now? Each time I'd choke. It was scary.

Some nurses got mad easily and said to forget about the machine. Forget about breathing in and out–just let the machine do it. It was hard because I would choke. Finally I learned not to breathe at all when I swallowed–just hold my breath and swallow–stop breathing and swallow. It was not easy to learn that, but already I was beginning. My first step in recovery was to learn how to breathe. The second step, how to swallow and the third, how to pee. Everything contained–in and out, in and out, in and out with the big yellow machine. It became warm and comforting. It embraced me utterly.

Barbara Williams was the nurse in that Isolation unit and Dr. Smith Peterson was the doctor. I was okay being there. I felt every detail of being alive then. My world suddenly had become extremely small and tight inside the machine, inside the room, cared for by individual people. I was very small and my whole world had suddenly become small, tight and precise. I paid attention to every tiny piece of life, as I watched the tan sponge rubber cuff puff out and get sucked in as I breathed in and out, in and out. And I took careful sips of water and juice. And I peed. All of that was very important. My world had gotten so very tiny and I was very small but, I was alive.

The Iron Lung was snug and comfortable and later when I spent time on the rocking bed, I would look forward to going back into it. The huge mechanical rocking bed was squeezed into the small hospital room, too. It looked like a regular hospital bed, except that it was on a platform rocker and when it was turned on it tilted up and down like a seesaw. The big yellow tank remained in the middle of the room with me in it most of the time. There were portholes on either side of it, so the nurses could reach in and provide care. On each side were two round portholes and on one side the opening was oblong so a bed pan could fit through. The nurses gave me a bath through the portholes or rolled me on my side and did the simple exercises needed to relieve the pain caused by muscle spasms. These were passive exercises where I would do nothing.

While I was in the Lung I felt detached from the rest of my body. My face (my head) was the only part of me outside the machine. The rest of me was inside and beyond me, out of my reach. I became more aware of my body when I came out of the Lung and got weaned onto the Rocking Bed, which was near the wall. The bed rocked deep. Head to toe. When the bed rocked deep to the head, I'd breathe in and when it rocked deep to the toe I'd breathe out. There was a rhythm. My head would go way down as my toes would come way up and then my toes would go way down as my head would come way up. At first I got a nose bleed when I was on the bed and the nurses put me back in the Lung. I felt wonderfully snug back in the lung–perfectly safe in there.

I was increasingly aware of my body when I was on the Rocking Bed.

Especially my hands–my right hand. I struggled to get my right hand up to my face. It took a few weeks, day after day, to make my hand inch its way up to my face. I wanted to touch my face–to scratch my itchy eyes.

When I got my hand to my chin I'd stick out my tongue and use my tongue to pull my hand all the way to my face. That was my very first feeling of accomplishment–achievement of having "done it." I was getting to know the physical therapists too. Every day, two sets of exercises were done several times. The passive exercises were for range of motion and kept my muscles stretched out, so they wouldn't contract and stay that way. Those were done after the hot packs were removed. The active exercises were for me to work as hard as I could to encourage muscles back to life–back to usefulness. There were very particular exercises for my hands and arms–each finger, thumb, wrist, elbow and shoulder. These exercises took a long time every morning and again every afternoon. My legs too–toes, ankles, knees and hips. It was hard work that took lots of concentration. I wanted my hands to work again. I wanted to feed myself. I wanted to hold the fork myself. When my breathing got strong enough, I stayed out of the Lung for longer periods of time. And eventually off the Rocking Bed, too. I began going to the pool for exercises. The pool was down stairs and Joe Brown would come up with a stretcher around 10:30 in the morning and bring me down there. The pool had an overhead rail from which hung canvas stretchers. Joe Brown would transfer me from one stretcher to the other and walk around the edge of the pool to where he'd lower it and me down to the physical therapist waiting in the water. The water felt wonderful. I especially liked Miss Cutting. She grew up in Chelsea, Massachusetts where Dad had been born. There were tables in the pool and all my exercises were done on those tables. My body felt light and would float.

Miss Bassett, Sally Bassett, was a physical therapist with another way of helping. She did electro therapy on the muscles of my hands. Her office was down the hall and three times a week I was taken to her on a stretcher. She had an instrument that looked like a silver pencil with a round gauze pad at one end and an electrical cord at the other end. Miss Bassett dipped the padded end in some water and placed it very carefully on my hand. The current made my hand tingle and the muscles responded as Miss Bassett coached me to bring my thumb "out around and over" and sure enough, with the help of the electrical stimulation my thumb did just what she and I together asked it to do. It all helped. The hot packs helped too. They smelled of wet wool and they got itchy when they cooled down. Several times a day the nurses rolled in the silver hot pack machine and pulled out the steaming, tan colored pieces of wet wool and quickly wrapped each leg and each arm with a hot pack. Then they covered each with a towel. Twenty minutes later they came back to remove the cold itchy packs. These kept muscles from tightening and contracting. There was great emphasis on keeping muscles limber. Many of the exercises became very painful as the muscles wanted to tighten and contract and the exercises kept them stretched out. After several months, when I no longer slept in the Iron Lung I slept at night with an airplane splint which kept my shoulder muscles stretched out. There was a board under my back and shoulders with wings on either side to rest my arms. My arms were strapped to the wings and sand bags were used to keep the wings extended. My Catholic school days made me think of Jesus on the Cross. At night I thought about that a lot. A little lady Jesus nailed to a cross. My legs were enclosed in plaster leg casts. All of this to keep my paralyzed body from contracting and becoming deformed. I remember crying softly when no one was around.

A Child of 10

A child of ten, I was–a child of ten. Ordinary. With freckles. Wearing blue overalls and sneakers. Always set and ready for surprises! And oh yes, surprises did come. New people. A new script. A whole new way of being in this world. I was ten one minute and ageless the next. I was standing tall and ready for anything one minute and the next minute I was paralyzed– unable to breathe, eat, roll over, pee or swallow my tears. My life had begun anew that day–anew in the big yellow tank–The Iron Lung. My cocoon. Finally, I was warm and safe and cared for.

I trusted those busy people in white rushing all around me–focusing on me. I was the center of the universe. I looked straight up into my oblong mirror and saw the whole world of my being–the doorway behind me and the nurses' station beyond the doorway. I whimpered and all their heads turned toward me. I pretended to whimper and they turned back to their 3:P.M. report. So I whimpered again–louder and they all turned again. Magic. I had magic. I really didn't need any one of them for the moment. I was just checking things out. They'd come soon enough anyway without me requesting them. They came in constantly–to see me–to look at me–to turn me over, feed me, give me a bed pan. Or to exercise my limp and unmoving limbs–limbs that were cut off from my view–limbs contained inside the yellow tank. Only my head moved from side to side. And my eyes. My eyes also moved a little–open and close, open and close. I could wiggle my nose and open my mouth and nod my head slightly. And because I was ten, I wasn't thinking about tomorrow and tomorrow and tomorrow. Enough for now are the surprises of today. And a surprise did come today–A Grand surprise!

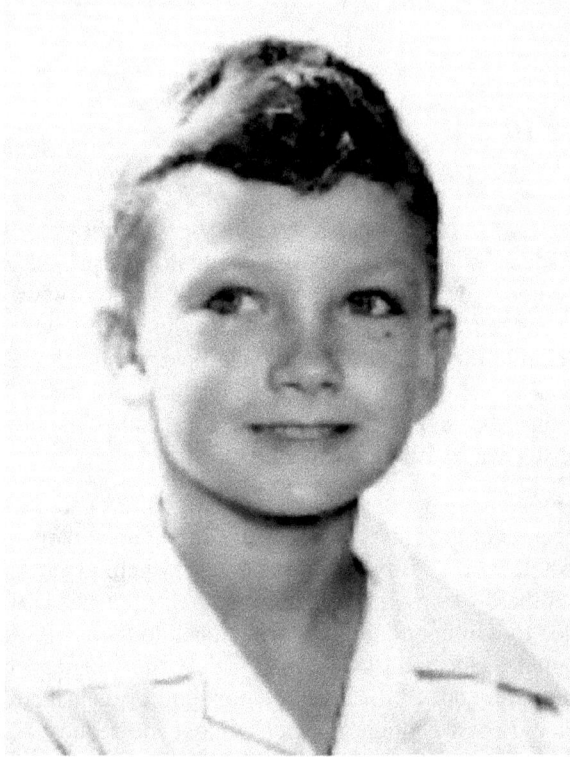

Jackie, age 10

Jackie came in to see me. I was so happy to see his familiar face–his normal face. And the main thing that surprised me? He looked at me normal and talked to me normal, like before. Nothing had changed in his eyes. I was still me to him! He stayed an hour until they made him leave. I love Jackie. He is more than a cousin to me. I told him I would be in a wheelchair when I got home. He told me that was good, because he would ride on it with me.

He did.

Miss Wentworth

As Miss Wentworth hurries about, the words of the song play over and over in my mind. "Only five minutes more... give me five minutes more."

She hurries to be off duty by eleven o'clock. I love having her work evenings like this, because we have more time informally together than when she works the day shift. On the day shift Miss Wentworth is Head Nurse. She is very busy and very serious because she has to keep a steady eye on all the student nurses. She makes sure everything is just so in Division 36. She tapes little hand written notes on the doors and walls and on the beds of her polio patients. Her crisp white uniform rustles as she walks quickly and purposefully from duty to duty. The square white hat that identifies her as a Children's Hospital Nursing School Graduate, sits on the back of her head framed by her dark curly hair. I love Miss Wentworth. I love having her fluttering around me. I always want more of her time.

I am on the Rocking Bed tonight, located beside the wall with the foot end of the bed near the door. I can see more from the Rocking Bed than I can in the Respirator. Now I can see down the hall. I can watch her coming and going as she does all the busy chores before she is finished for the night. I watch as she leaves–calling out "Good Night" for the third and forth time. And the words of the song stay in my head... "Five minutes more, give me five minutes more."

Miss Wentworth has a wonderful way of looking right at you. She looks into my face–straight into my face, as if she really and truly wants to see me. She smiles easily and I feel loved. She frowns and I see how worried she is because I didn't eat. She scoops me up under my arms and under my knees and transfers me from my bed to the stretcher, waiting to take me somewhere else–to X-Ray, or the Pool, or The Plaster Room. I wait there on the stretcher in the hallway and watch her as she hurries about. An Orderly will usually come for me and return me later. But if Miss Wentworth is still on duty she'll come back, scoop me up in her arms again and return me to my bed.

Division 36 was a busy Polio Unit and Miss Wentworth kept it running efficiently. She had only the Supervisor, Miss Kerr, to answer to. Miss Kerr regularly inspected everything and Miss Wentworth wanted to make sure that everything met with her approval. And most often it did. If Miss Kerr found the tiniest thing out of order she would make sure Miss Wentworth felt her disapproval. She wore the square Children's Hospital cap, too. One time Miss Kerr noticed with a critical look on her face that there was not a salt or pepper shaker on my lunch tray and Miss Wentworth commented that it wasn't necessary anyway because a child's taste buds were not developed and didn't need seasoning. I thought she was crazy. But no one got in trouble over the absence of the salt and pepper shaker.

Miss Wentworth took very good care of me. I believe I was her favorite. Even though she was the Head Nurse, lots of times she took personal care of me. She gave me my bath and transferred me from the Respirator to the Rocking Bed and kept an eye on me to see that I was okay. She fed me lots of times and continued to worry because I ate so little.

And there was Dorothy Shea the Cleaning Lady. She wore a blue uniform with a white apron and every morning she came in to dust and clean my room. Dorothy talked to me about herself and her daughter, Ida. I liked her and she liked me too. She made Cream of Wheat for me, which I did like to eat. And Irene Cutting liked me and so did Dr. Grice and Miss McGinnis. They liked me because I worked very hard and I wasn't a cry baby. Lots of people really liked me on Division 36 and I really liked them. One night in August there was a thunder and lightening storm and the electricity went off. And so did my Iron Lung! The nurses hurried to grab the pump at the other end of the tank and one by one they took turns manually pumping the Lung! Suddenly Dr. Banks ran into the room all excited because he had ripped a hole in his pants jumping over a fence in his effort to get to us and help pump the Lung! It wasn't long before the electricity came back on and everyone relaxed! I had begun to have a whole new life on Division 36 and I felt even more and more distant from Ma and Dad as my former life at home began to fade into the background.

In the Fall, Miss Wentworth went on vacation for a long weekend to her parents' home in Holden, Mass. a little town outside of Worcester and she asked me what I wanted her to bring back–I said, "Apples." And she did. She brought back a whole bag of apples. I loved those apples!

I was hospitalized again and again in the immediate years following the onset of Polio and Miss Wentworth was always there as a comfort. One time, late in the day, when I was sitting in my wheelchair near the Nurses' station, Miss Wentworth and I were talking. She took my hand in both of her hands and kissed my fingers. Her love was a blessing that I held in my consciousness as I traveled through darkened corridors during the next few years. She told me about her boyfriend, Ken. I thought Ken was lucky to have Miss

Wentworth for his girlfriend. When they were married in May 1952 Miss Wentworth wanted me to be at her Wedding. She asked me to be in charge of her Guest Book. I wore a soft green dress with a corsage of tiny pink roses. It was a big occasion for me and for Ma and Dad too because Dad had to drive all the way to Holden and it was more of an outing than we had imagined possible since I had Polio.

All in all, knowing Miss Wentworth made Division 36 and my new life as a polio patient special.

Homeward Bound

On May 4th I left Division 36. I was Discharged to go home to Ma, Dad, Peggy and Paul. The only time Peggy and Paul came to see me in the Hospital was on Christmas Day. I really only missed Paul who was three years old when I got home and some of our neighbors didn't want their children to play with him, because they thought he'd give them my Polio. Ma said Peggy cried when I got sick. She wanted me to be okay. Ma said Dad cried, too. She said that at the kitchen table at breakfast, the day after I was hospitalized, Dad said "If anything happens to her that's the end of me." In those days no one directly cared for the stricken family members. Ma had got a job at Whitmore's Greenhouses to take her mind off of the "tragic" thing that had happened to our family, but now she had to give that up.

Riding home in the front seat of the Plymouth between Ma and Dad, I was terrified of the traffic as Dad drove through the unfamiliar Boston streets. Also, I was worried that Ma might resent me for having to give up her job, or that her migraine headaches might make her unable to take care of me like what happened two times on my weekend visits home, when Ma got so sick she had to go to bed and Mrs. Elliott came over and took care of me. No one at the Hospital knew about that because Ma told me not to tell them.

But at last we finally made it safely home and Dad pulled the car into the garage. He carried me through the cellar and up the ten narrow stairs through the kitchen to my new bedroom, which used to be Ma's lovely dining room, but from now on would be my new hospital room. My bed was set where Ma's lovely table used to be. Dad put the solid mahogany table down the cellar along with her highly polished mahogany buffet. A folding screen separated the dining room from the living room so I would have privacy using the bed pan and having a bed bath.

Ma's friend, Winnie Russell, gave us a small TV with a seven inch screen, which Dad fixed up with a 12 inch magnifier and when the screen was open, me and Jackie could watch it all the way from my bed. We would watch the half hour soap opera, Hawkins Falls and Kate Smith who opened every show singing "God Bless America."

An Uncle To Be Disremembered

After eight months in the Iron Lung, I had come home from Children's Hospital to face two severely unwanted visitors, Aunt Alice and Uncle Mike. Alice was reconciled with Ma for a while and they would regularly come to our house to visit. Aunt Alice would be loaded down with sweet pastries from the Supreme Bakery in Lynn and cigars for Dad—treats that really weren't treats. We couldn't enjoy them because there were grandiose feelings attached to the treats that we had to acknowledge, that made Aunt Alice shine so wonderfully special and generous to a fault for bringing all those treats that none of us really wanted. There were feelings between her and Ma, they made believe weren't there—feelings and thoughts they tried so hard to cover up with banal chatter. It never worked.

And then there was lechery personified in Uncle Mike. I hadn't forgotten his earlier invasion of my privacy and dignity at 16 Perley St. but the difference was, I could no longer run away like I had done in Lynn. Peggy hated him as much as I did. He would grab Peggy and kiss her mouth and she'd pull away and leave the room. No one appeared to notice. If they did, no one said anything.

He wasn't in our house for more than a half hour, when he sat by my bed, reached under the covers and touched the private parts of my body. It was all happening again. I was frozen stiff, horrified, but no one noticed and I felt awful—ashamed and small. Scared to death, I called out to Ma and Dad for something—anything, "Water," or "Adjust my pillow Ma, *please*." anything to bring them back into my view. And when they would come in, Uncle Mike just stood up and stretched like everything was normal and strolled back into the living-room. I told Ma I didn't want to be left alone with Uncle Mike. I told her I didn't like him.

Ma said we couldn't say anything because we'd hurt Aunt Alice's feelings, so I should not be a trouble maker. So I stayed scared, small and defenseless. Ma and Dad didn't like Mike either, but the thought of him doing anything like that was utterly out of their realm of possibilities or comprehension. A world of that nature did not exist for either one of them. So when Uncle Mike would come by, there was no relief from the awfulness of his presence. He would sit near me when no one was around and if he didn't touch me he'd talk about touching me. I froze up–held myself tight and small inside my barbed wire cage. I felt dirty. It was like before polio, with Timmy. There was some awful thing about me. And it was a secret. It was always a secret. Worst of all there was something about it that I liked—the way I liked the feelings I had in my body long ago when I played naked in the woods with Timmy. When we played together like we knew we shouldn't. When we touched each other's bodies and looked at each other's body alone in the woods. Secret. And Uncle Mike found me again–even in my home-hospital bed, he found me and I couldn't get away from him or myself to be safe. Uncle Mike made me feel dirty all over again. And I had thought Polio had rescued me from myself. But no, not even Polio rescued me then.

After Dad moved my bed farther over, toward the door, so I could look through the dining-room into the living-room and watch the TV. I could hardly believe it when Timmy Kimbal showed up unannounced one evening. I hadn't seen him since before Polio. He bragged about being the greatest baseball player around and we watched TV for a while. Dad and Peggy were out and Ma was taking a bath upstairs. Timmy was sitting beside my bed and wasn't there long before he moved his hand under the sheet and found a way to touch me. He showed me what happened to his penis when he shook it and it got big and stiff and hard and white stuff came out of it. He wanted me to shake it and make the white stuff come out of it.

I was scared, but felt excited too. I wanted to run away and hide. But I couldn't. There was no way I could escape from myself and no one I could talk to. I was all alone in my room, in my house, in my barbed wire cage. All locked up–small, afraid, defiled, PARALYZED! No girlfriend to tell. The public image of a sick child. As Lee Hussey would say, "Our sweet little polio girl," That's what I was on the outside to everyone–"a sweet little polio girl," at twelve, thirteen and fourteen.

Somewhere along the way, Ma and Aunt Alice had a falling out and I finally got rid of Uncle Mike. Ma and Aunt Alice didn't reconcile again until after Mike died. And Timmy grew older and didn't come around anymore. All my bad feelings stayed locked inside of me and all the while I pretended to be the sweet little polio girl, still scared.

1951

It was summer again, only 1951 and I was almost twelve. Jackie hung out with me almost every day. He sat by my bed and he let me play with his hair which felt smooth and silky almost. We watched the new console television given to us by Frank McGovern and some of the other men Dad worked with. Frank delivered it to us and he cried when he talked to me. He couldn't stop the tears from streaming down his face. Jackie and I thought that was kind of weird. I was able to sit up in my wheelchair for an hour in the morning and an hour in the afternoon. But I was confined to the house because there were several steps to go out our back door and to go out the front door there were the wooden stairs leading down from the porch and the cement steps from there to the sidewalk. Ma couldn't get me in or out by herself. "Confined," was the way she phrased it. She would say Barbara is "confined" to the wheelchair and I learned more of what the word meant by the way it felt when Ma spoke it.

Somehow the men on the Stoneham Fire Department found out about me and they decided to offer their help and friendship. When I wanted to go outside, one of the Firemen would come down and carry first my chair and then me outside. Jackie liked to push me in my chair. He would push me up to Stoneham Square to Grants and the 5 & 10 cent store which were a half mile from Cottage St. and after we finished looking at stuff, Jackie would ride on the back of the chair down the hills back home which was scary but great fun. When we got there, Ma would call the Firemen and another fellow would come over and help me back into the house. Sometimes when we needed a ride to the Polio Clinic at Children's Hospital, a Fireman drove us all the way into Boston. Bill Meehan was my favorite and Bob O'Melia was also a really nice guy. All the others were nice, too. At Christmas they would bring me a gift. One Christmas they gave me a Vanity Table with a mirror and Mrs. Elliott made a fluffy, feminine skirt for it.

Dad was home on weekends and would carry me down through the cellar to the car and take me over to Malden for Physical Therapy. The clinic was on Main Street among all the interesting small stores that I liked looking at from the car window and Dad's arms as he carried me in from the car. He would lay me down on a hard table and the Therapist lady would do a series of stretching exercises to prevent the muscle contractions and a series of active exercises to strengthen recovering muscles, much like they did at Children's Hospital. Ma would come with us and stand by to help if the Therapy lady needed assistance. Some Physical Therapists were really good at their job and I knew when I had a good one, because of the sure way she held my body and bent me as far to one side as she could until I couldn't stand the sharp pain in my side any longer and she would skillfully release the action for a moment and then bend my body again and again and again. Ten times this way and then she would move to the other side of the table and bend my body ten times the other way. And I knew for sure she was really good when she was not too timid to allow me to feel as much pain as I could tolerate. And silently, I would pray and think about Jesus and how much his side must have hurt when one of the soldiers pierced his side with a spear when he was on the cross. I would think and think and think again and again of that and as I did the pain in my side lessened–lightened up slightly. It didn't go away, but it finally got bearable. Then she would do stretching exercises on both of my legs and arms and perform the active exercises. It took about a half hour and when we were done Dad carried me back to the car and we drove home. Many times on that ride back my vision would become blurred and by the time we got home I had a wicked headache over my right eye that didn't quit for hours, until I got sick and threw up and finally would get some relief in sleep.

For about three years, we continued to make that trip to Malden on Saturday mornings, and later on it was in a small room in an Elementary School building. At those times they would put heavy, black, iron leg braces on me with heavy leather straps that attached to the plastic body cast I wore. With all of that on me they would stand me up beside the exercise table to practice holding my balance. With Canadian Crutches on each arm I would lean to my left and then to my right. Eventually, by gravity rather than strength, my leg came forward and because I leaned on it, my other leg came forward and I stepped out as though walking. We would work that way for a half hour until I was all tired out. Then Ma would take the braces off and Dad would drive us home again–me still between them on the front seat of the Plymouth–that same gray Plymouth that had taken us to Island Falls.

At twelve and a half, my former classmates at St. Pat's were in the 7th grade and that strange experience of having "my friend" happened to me. Bleeding. staining. "Every month," Ma said, "From now on, it means that you can have a baby. And that's the blood that would make a baby, but if you're not having a baby the blood must come out every month." Hearing all of that, I lapsed into a state of shock and felt stupid and ashamed. Everyone else knew more than I knew about it, so I pulled myself deep inside of me to hide–paralyzed in my bed in the dining room.

I didn't know what to ask for anymore. I didn't know what I needed or wanted. Ma was all worn out and I went limp. I was fed, bathed and given a bedpan, wiped clean, dressed, picked up and put into my wheelchair. I felt dead. And adding to it, I had that uninvited "friend" every month. I was dead and bleeding.

None of it made any sense to me. I weighed 42 pounds and my whole life transpired in three rooms–the living room, the kitchen and in Ma's dining room that had become my bedroom. I lived all of it in those three rooms, or in my wheelchair. But my mind kept me connected to Children's Hospital, which was my main connection to the outside world. I REALLY lived THERE. I was connected to Miss Wentworth, Dr. Grice and Miss McGinnis–connected to all the activity of that place. I would rather have been there, even though I wasn't supposed to rather be there. I was supposed to rather be at home, but I felt scared there at home–having to make myself fit back into that bizarre world around me again. So I pulled myself in, tighter and tighter in that miniscule world–their little world–unable to alter any of it–even for one blessed moment. My only control or power was to burrow deeper and deeper into myself, and watch. It is all so clear to me today. I didn't cry. I hardly ever cried. I smiled. I was supposed to smile. Ann Lee called me, "Our sweet little Polio girl." So, so clear to me: Ma is disheveled. Her stockings are twisted with runs in them. Her housedress is torn under the arm and her apron is soiled. She rolls her hair and holds it in place with hairpins. All my feelings hardened and hid. Ma went blindly from task to endless task–not feeling. All her rage buried so deep and only released when she fought with Peggy. All Ma's anger exploded in blind fury when Peggy behaved like her fifteen year old self. Ma screamed out–a screeching, horrible tirade directed at Peggy whose face became frozen in resentment and hatred. Dad took off his belt and Peggy cowered in the kitchen against the cabinets until Ma broke through her own screaming rage to stop Dad from hitting Peggy with his belt. Peggy walked away. Ma retreated. Dad went limp in his chair. I stayed still–five paralyzed people living together, but I was the only one labeled "the victim." Yes I was the Polio "Victim" but constantly reminded that there were five paralyzed, stricken "victims"–all labeled differently. Peggy was labeled "difficult and selfish," I was labeled "the sweet little polio girl." Paul was labeled "a good boy." Dad was silent, a hard worker–a good man." Ma was the "devout, obedient martyr."

The polio virus stays in your body only a few days, but that brief period it is there, it damages your body so badly that you know it can be none other than forever. Yes, it is forever. The Polio is gone and paralysis remains. So we follow Doctor's Order's, doggedly docile and submissive, like we follow the Ten Commandments and the Rules of the Catholic Church.

Father Burke came to the house each week to bring me Holy Communion. Ma met him at the front door with a lighted candle and she confessed to him that my fast had been broken because I had taken a drink of water during the night. He went away and did not give me Communion because I had taken the water. I felt scared most of the time and mostly it affected my stomach–filling me up so that I couldn't eat. My tongue pressed feverishly tight against the roof of my mouth, keeping nourishment out and pain in. Silent paralysis. Life went on around me and I watched. Life happened to me and I stayed very still. There was no point in struggling against it because that only hurt more. Like a trapped animal. The more it rails against the trap the more it hurts. So the animal goes limp, stays still, to avoid the pain. Peggy directs her anger openly toward Ma, Dad, Me and Paul and in return she gets all of Ma's rage directed toward her. It drives her deeper and deeper into her own simmering fury. She breaks loose from it and screams angry words at me. No one, no counselor, teacher or friend, sits down with Peggy who is fifteen to ask what she makes of it all. No one sits with Paul who is four or Ma or Dad. We all go on in the darkness not knowing each other or ourselves.

I have one thread of life leading me out of this hell and that is solely my connection to Children's Hospital. I keep my eye on Miss Wentworth. I love her and she loves me. Dr. Grice is smart and knows what to do. He can get me through this. There is a tremendous power in him. I do everything he tells me to do. I watch him. Every six weeks we go to the Polio Clinic, Ma and me, and when we get home we follow his orders.

And Jackie and I continued to share that other world–that TV world inhabited by Roy Rogers, Dale Evans, The Lone Ranger, Hopalong Cassidy, The Texaco Show with Uncle Milty. And on Sundays, the Ed Sul-livan "Shew" and at eight o'clock on Friday (fish day) "I Remember Mama" was brought to us by *Maxwell House Coffee* (good til the last drop).

Summer has arrived early this year
I sleep with only a sheet
I feel good
I am refreshed
When I awake early–at pre-dawn
I hear the birds–loud and insistent
rousing one another
They say, "Here I am'
"Come with me"
And they call to me, too
They say, "A new day is dawning -
Wake up! -
There are things to do this day!
Don't let it slip away! -
Get up and be ALIVE today!"

Twelve and a Half

Yes I am twelve and a half, but I was paralyzed at age ten and all of my life had stopped right there. I seemed destined to remain forever a child under the stationary umbrella of age ten–Dad's little Stevie. And for Ma, I was a magnet–an unrelenting, insistent call to come out of her daydream, to come away from her reverie, to pay absolute attention to the needs of her sick child. And even further for Ma, my Polio meant migraine headaches. Out of her introversion so desperately concealed, she resisted with migraines and words that said, "No, no, not now, not NOW!" Time was not right–never right for thrusting her out of her reverie–out of that private place where she was safe. Polio made Ma unsafe. Polio pulled Ma out of her hide-a-way world. Polio exposed Ma and she hated it and resented me immensely for it all. And poor Dad. He was so sad. He went to work every day and came home every night at quarter to five. He'd pat my head. "How are you doing, Stevie?" he'd say to the boy he yearned for–the boy he would never hunt and fish with. They grieved alone–separated by a massive wall of concrete in the solitude of their separate lives. Their twin beds separated their twin grief. They lived separate and alone from each other–separate and alone from their children. And their children lived separate and alone from them and from each other. Ma and Dad kept up appearances. They were strong. They kept a stiff upper lip. They dried secret tears. They kept the Faith. They kept right on going, kept going, going, going on... and on...

Aunt Nora, who was seventy-five in 1950, was around a lot in those years. She would bring along countless stories about other people who had Polio. She would say to me, "Go kick a football Tenley. Tenley Albright had Polio and look at her now. She's a world champion Ice Skater!" Ma would respond wearily and say, "Aunt Nora, there's Polio and then there's Polio. Some get it worse than others." Aunt Nora didn't have room in her mind for that information. To her, Polio was Polio! Some people got it and fought harder than others. The ones that fought harder got better. The one's that didn't fight hard enough didn't get better. "Franklin Delano Roosevelt had Polio and he became President of the United States!" And Aunt Nora would continue to tell me numerous stories about people worse off than me–stories she had read about in the Boston newspapers, or *Reader's Digest*. The best story of all, was the story about a man who needed to have hip surgery that would fuse his hips one way or the other, so he had to decide if he wanted to sit or stand for the rest of his life! That was Aunt Nora's ultimate "worse off" story. With her bad hearing, she would lean over my wheelchair and yell into my face: "Would you rather sit or stand for the rest of your life?" But I was never offended because I knew that Aunt Nora liked me a lot and she meant well. I tried not to laugh at her and I'd answer, "I don't know, Aunt Nora but gee, that's awful. I really didn't know!" And so she would tell me in detail, the whole story all over again. Years later after Aunt Nora had passed away, it became kind of a family joke. From time to time, when things seemed to get tougher and tougher, or when we heard a depressing story, or our own story got pretty tough, Ma would say, "For Heaven's sake, would you rather sit or stand for the rest of your life?" And that would lighten things up a little. Aunt Nora was okay. She didn't know anymore than anybody else what to do about all that Polio! It was like that. People telling stories. Legends. Movie stars who had Polio. Helen Hayes' daughter died from Polio. For those who survived Polio there was a "halo" for them. If you had Polio, you must find a way to shine. The smartest or the prettiest or the most popular. That's how people tried to make it be okay. The reality was different. I wasn't the smartest, or the prettiest, or the most popular. I was ordinary and a lot of the time, I felt less than ordinary. I was a ten year old child. Quiet and shy. I worked hard–worked hard and tired easily. And I was constantly warned against fatigue. Fatigue was the number one enemy. Just don't get fatigued! Somehow Ma and Dad really heard that warning and saw to it that I didn't push myself into fatigue! "Stop before you get fatigued!" "Stop before you get over tired!" "Stop! Stop! Stop!" The message I heard was "STOP!"

Yes the outside me stopped–the me that liked to ride Peggy's blue bike–the me that liked the snow and sledding and the me that looked forward to vacationing again at Island Falls. On the outside, all of me stopped. But the inside of me did not stop. I stayed small and hidden. But I did not stop. My inner landscape did not stop growing. My body-life that encased me, stopped. I did not stop. I watched. I watched Ma and I watched Peggy and Jackie's sister, cousin Bette Jean. I watched Connie Elliott growing and enlarging her life and Beadie Vierra, across the street, always going somewhere. I watched Ma dress Peggy up for high school and I watched as Peggy got to be pretty and popular. I watched her dress up for her dates and her proms. I watched as Peggy became the prettiest and the most popular girl in the neighborhood. And the most popular girl in the High School. And Bette Jean became Queen of the Winter Carnival Ball. Ma and Aunt Dot lived their desperate lives through their daughters, Peggy Ann and Bette Jean, while Jackie and I watched. Jackie got stuck back there, too. We both got stuck. We knew it and we stuck together!   103

At home my world consisted of Ma and Dad, Peggy, Paul, Jackie, Mrs. Elliott and my home tutor, Mrs. Heath. I loved Paul and enjoyed Jackie. Once a month I went in to the Polio Clinic at Children's Hospital. Transportation was sometimes a problem when the Firemen would be out on calls and Dad had to work. For a while, the Red Cross sent volunteers–women, who would drive us into Boston. One was Mrs. Herson–a sweet white haired lady. I really liked her. Once, on the way home we stopped at a Car-Hop on Memorial Drive in Cambridge for lunch. The waitress came out to the car on roller skates, took our order and brought the food on a tray that attached to the car window. I had grilled cheese and a root beer. There was another Red Cross lady that I did not like at all. I forget her name. There was one thing I especially disliked about her. She used to lift me in and out of the car and when she did she slipped her hand under me and touched between my legs. I wanted to scream, jump up and run away, the way I ran away in Lynn when Uncle Mike touched me like that. I hated her, but I said nothing. Ma was always so effusively grateful for the ride. But I really cringed when I overheard Aunt Dot say, "She is such a lovely lady. I was so touched when I saw the caring way she treats Barbara." A lovely lady, indeed.

Other women from the Parish would come to the house to visit me. They were called The Legion of Mary. I didn't like them or their visits. They just came and sat beside my bed and said nothing. Ma didn't know what to do with them. She didn't know if she was supposed to feed them, talk to them, or just let them sit there beside my bed. Jackie and I thought they were funny. I was supposed to be nice and polite to them. Ma thought they were nosey. After a while they would finally get up and leave. I felt relief when they left. So did Ma and so did Jackie. They were an intrusion and an interruption. At Christmas the Girl Scouts came and stood around my hospital bed and sang Christmas Carols. Jackie and I couldn't stop giggling and in the kitchen Ma couldn't stop crying.

Fourteen

The year I turned fourteen I was in bed from July until the following March–all wrapped up in the total body cast and Ma took complete care of me. She brought me my meals. She bathed me and brought me the bed pan. It was hard to grow up. It was hard to grow my body up all wrapped up in Plaster-of-Paris like that. It was hard to grow up having Ma doing all those things for me every day. I stayed all wrapped up on the outside. On the inside I continued to watch and pay attention.

In the hospital, when Doctor Grice was making decisions about my spinal fusion, my body became disgustedly public. My body had to be studied–looked at, X-rayed and photographed over and over, again and again. One time they laid me on the floor, with all of my clothes removed, on my stomach, to photograph my back. I was terrified and humiliated, but was grateful that Dr. Grice was there. He placed me on the floor, stayed close by me and kept his hand on my arm, although he said nothing directly to me, but I was relieved that he didn't let go of me. Other times they wanted to take pictures of me sitting up. I had no balance, no trunk stability and no control over my body remaining upright, so when they sat me up, they supported my body with sandbags and pillows and took more pictures. I tried to separate myself from myself. My eyes stung and my tongue pressed hard against the roof of my mouth, but all I really did was push my fear and humiliation down deeper and deeper and deeper, until I was buried deep, deep inside of myself. I lived deep, deep inside that shell of myself–a shell that had stopped being me. I was way down deep inside that barbed wire cage. What showed on the outside was a smile, a brave smile without words. All the words were buried with me, inside, way down deep inside. I buried all my words and people said I was quiet. "Quiet, shy, and pretty, too" that's how my classmates described me in our High School class yearbook years later in 1959.

There were days of emptiness when I needed to fold myself all up, to reduce the pain somehow, but could not. There was no relief–no way out, resulting in a state of unknowingness born out of its own darkness and carried out in darkness–a self-engineered conspiracy along with the outward intrusive pressures to infantilize me–to keep me forever a sick child, needing others to care for my every need and in every instance, to protect me. I would instantly squash those feelings so desperate to emerge and find facile and practical reasons why I would forgive on the spot, yes analyzing and trying to understand, but not through the reality of feelings, but by intellectualizing everything and burying alive the true reality of what I was experiencing. Day by day I compromised myself more and more and incrementally drifted further into that state of unknowingness, denying carte blanche what I was feeling and what I truly wanted and needed to express or say. Instead, so as not to feel too deeply, I kept my breathing shallow and stayed on the surface, denying the emptiness below, leaving all that agony cut off, to dwell in utter aloneness, fear and despair below the throat, which I held tight with a death grip. My throat stayed shut tight against all that egregious and hurtful turmoil, holding back the haunting memories of "Go away, Don't come close, We don't want you here..." I lived that way day by day, by day, by endless days to be followed by... endless nights.

Mrs. Elliott was Ma's best friend–as good a next door neighbor a neighbor could possibly be. Ma would say, "She knows how to solve problems. If you have a problem, Helen Elliott will sit down with you and think it through. She will think about it until the problem is solved." Sometimes Mrs. Elliott would go home before the problem was solved. Later she would appear at the back door with a solution.

Ma depended on Mrs. Elliott. She was Ma's teacher. Her daughter Connie was just a baby when Ma and Dad were first married and had moved to Cottage Street. The Elliott's had two other children at the time–Eileen and Doris. Ma got pregnant with Peggy soon after she was married and Connie gave her a good model for developmental points of comparison, but Peggy, being so much like Peggy was, the comparison was not often a favorable one.

Mrs. Elliott never wore make-up. Ma said she looked matronly.

She was a seamstress and made lots of Connie's clothes. She did laundry, cooking, cleaning and sewing at home and also worked hard for the Church. In the summers, Ma and Mrs. Elliott would talk over the fence by the clothes line for hours. They would discuss "Confidential Chat," a homemakers column that appeared daily in the Boston Globe, which consisted of letters sent in under pen names from homemakers. Many of the letters were controversial and much different from the way Ma thought about things and she was almost certain that Mrs. Elliott wrote some of those letters and seemed to relish knowing that possible secret.

Mrs Elliott encouraged Ma to let me do things. She told Ma to let me help in the kitchen, but Ma said I couldn't help because my left arm wasn't strong enough and it was easier for her to do things herself. I felt safe with Mrs. Elliott. Many days she took me out with her when she went up town–pushed me in my metal chair and took me into all the stores. Ma wasn't comfortable pushing me out of doors. It made her self-conscious and ashamed of my Polio–felt she was to blame, although she knew she wasn't. She would tell me over and over again, how the doctors told her that there was nothing they could do to stop the Polio. Once I had it that was it. It needed to run its course. She couldn't let go of the tormenting thought that if only she had taken me to the hospital sooner–done something different, sooner. If only Dr. Burke had not been on vacation. But no. The doctors said, "No." It wouldn't have made any difference. Ma felt responsible just the same. How was she ever to know that Polio was a good thing that happened to me? How was anyone ever to know? But then, how could she ever know. That was *my* precious secret–not hers. Mrs. Elliott, Doris and Connie were good friends to me. Doris came over to curl my hair on Saturday afternoons before she went out on her dates with Georgie Bohling. She had a job as a secretary in Boston and earned $50.00 a week. Eventually Doris broke up with Georgie and married Ray. Connie liked to take me out with her. She liked to push me in my wheelchair. Ma said "Connie likes the attention it brings to her, unlike Peggy who didn't ever take Barbara out because she didn't want that sort of attention." Ma thought Connie was bold. Connie was in the Drum and Bugle Corp and took me to the Exhibition at Recreation Park in the summer. She met Johnny Kelly and loved him more than anyone in the world. They got married and had seven kids. The last two were twins.

Needed to see "What condition my condition was in."[1]

I remember those first days dawning, the awakening awareness of paralysis–the anvil-like total heaviness and inability to move independently. The solid immovable mass at ages of ten, twelve and still at sixteen–twisted, broken and heavy. Unable to move the whole of me, to raise myself up, or go from one place to another. The frightening awareness of my immobility, a solid mass needing to be moved only by the will, dedication and imposed duty of others–most usually Ma–the very one who needed Doctor's Orders to hold her infant until the baby turned red in the sun. Even when my body was simply that of a tiny doll girl, Ma needed to push me away so she could get on with her chores and her memories. Did she fear loving me? I have come to believe over the years that was so. And that's how I learned to talk myself out of and away from the feelings that created those sharp, piercing stomach pains–feelings of anger and sadness, fear and hurt–the muffled weeping and wailing congealing into pain that eventually refracted into emptiness. My stomach screamed at me to feel–screamed at me to feel all the anger and remorse of being paralyzed as a child and throughout adolescence and young adulthood–to scream out the lost dreams never experienced, good or bad. To scream the absence of the usual every day child struggles, replacing them with the unjustified demands of a twisted, broken body–too heavy for a young girl to manage herself and too ugly for her to invite someone else to manage it for her–to return to infancy at age ten, needing to be fed, bathed and toileted–lifted, dressed and pushed about in a carriage. In the summer when I was almost twelve, I wanted so much to lay on the grass–just to lay on the grass. So Ma and Mrs. Elliott did that for me. They lifted me out of the wheelchair and lay me down on the grass next to Dad's garden, near the apple tree I was no longer able to climb and I was where I thought I wanted to be, until I found I was alone and scared, because I couldn't move. I called to Ma and told her I would rather sit in my wheelchair. My world was no longer the way it was. My world was becoming Ma's Sister Christina's World.

I thought and thought and thought: How can I live inside this twisted broken body? My feet do things I don't want them to do. My ankles roll over

---

[1] (The First Edition, 1968) song written by Ricky Newbury

into uncomfortable positions. My feet don't lay flat on the foot pieces of the wheelchair. I am self-conscious of all the brokenness that I am. I am angry because Ma and Dad take care of me out of *their* brokenness–out of *their* frail, shattered spirits. *Their* sadness and grief incorporated into mine. I see my own despair reflected in their behavior toward me–in Dad's protectiveness–in Ma's determination to do what has to be done no matter what. She is locked into martyrdom. Dad is simply crushed and brokenhearted. I am still Stevie to him–his pal. But I am broken and can't be mended. I have to live the way I am. Jackie saw it and sang it to me in a low and kindly tone, "Stevie Duffy had a great fall and all the King's horses and all the King's men couldn't put Stevie Duffy together again."

Dad took good and gentle care of me–always. Weeks before he died, he was seventy-six and I was thirty-five. He laid a hand on my shoulder as he walked past me and murmured almost to himself, "I don't want to leave you." His gentleness was painful for me to see and accept. He was never tough, never demanding. His was a sad and gentle presence. Ma had turned her broken heart to stone years and years before Polio came into our lives. Polio was just one more reason to stay frozen and locked away. They were not there to comfort each other, or for healing, or for strength. And neither were emotionally present for Peggy when she was fourteen or Paul when he was three.

Yes, there were five broken hearts in our house then. And none of us knew how to come together to share the pain or heal the broken hearts. We each crawled into our own private selves and got lost. When Peggy was fifteen she found Paul Murphy and she clung to him for safety and strength. When brother Paul was in high school he found the Missionary life and escaped into the safety of Mill Hill and later the Maryknoll Fathers. Dad stayed gentle and sad. Ma stayed strong, the valiant warrior–the martyred mother carrying her cross– her burden to bear for this life.

There seemed to be no way out. I thought I had to somehow hold our family together. Even if Independent Living had been available to me then, I wonder if I would have been emotionally available to take advantage of it. There was a strong symbiotic relationship at home. I needed to keep Ma and Dad glued together. Somehow I thought if I was not at home the whole place would come unglued, fall apart, disappear. I thought there'd be no one there if I was not there. So I stayed paralyzed–immobilized by fear as well as by disease–fear that if I moved an inch the frail structure of our family would collapse. My solidness, my immobility, kept it all glued together. Somewhere deep inside of me I held that intuited, unspoken, belief and /or pet idea or feeling that Holden Caulfield wasn't the only "Catcher in the Rye."

North Truro

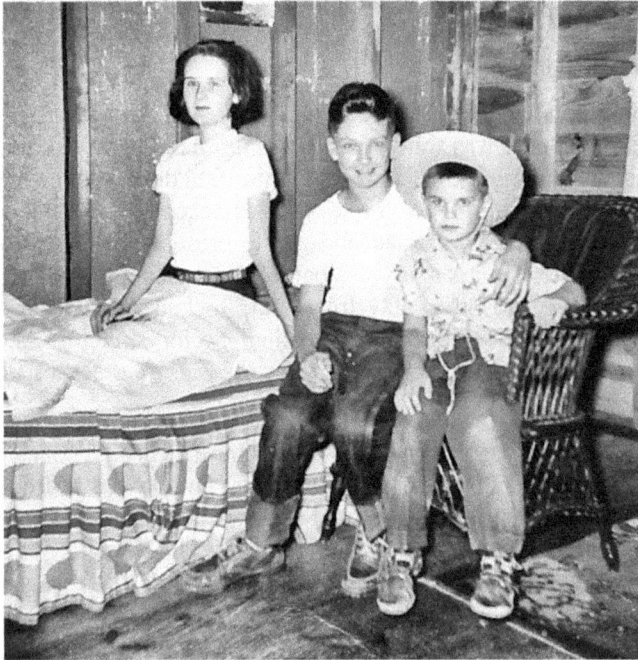

Barbara Jackie Paul

   It was in the summer of 1952. I was about to turn thirteen and I first read *The Catcher in the Rye*. We spent one week of Dad's vacation at North Truro on Cape Cod. At that time, North Truro was mostly dunes of sand, sea grass and water. Dad's friend, Bill Brookings, owned two cottages built high on the dunes overlooking the water and Dad rented one of them. Our cottage had brown weathered shingles and you could see the Pilgrim Monument at Provincetown from the back door. It was a Cape Cod cottage–boxlike, with single windows and flower boxes. The sea grass was tall green and brown around the cottage, sprouting up out of the sandy soil. There were only a few other cottages around then and only a handful of other people. Paul was five that summer and he thought Jackie was Superman. I was skinny and childlike in my body and dependent on Ma and Dad for everything. I wore the plaster body cast to keep my back straight while I sat in the wheelchair. Ma, who had fair complexion, didn't like the beach and chose to stay back at the cottage alone, while the rest of us headed for the water. And Jackie was with us–it was Dad, me, Paul, Jackie and Peggy. Peggy was sixteen and had been going with Paul Murphy for a while. Paul was from Lynn, Mass. and spent the weekends with us. The sky was blue and cloudless. The beach was endless–clean and empty. The waves rolled in from different directions all at the same time. Provincetown curled its tip out and around creating a sense of protection from the elements and seclusion. I went to the Beach with Dad, Peggy Paul and Jackie. Peggy held Paul in the water, teaching him how to swim. She was a strong swimmer. Ma said she too had been a strong swimmer when she was a girl, before she met Dad. Dad carried a heavy chaise lounge down to the beach which was about two hundred and fifty feet from the cottage–no small task. Then he would go back up and lug me down too. He'd stretched me out on it and then lie down on a large towel next to me, between taking dips in the ocean. Dad didn't call himself a strong swimmer–just a *good* swimmer taking long regular strokes as he lay on his back in the waves, always swimming across the water–never straight out. We stayed on the beach too long that day–just as Dad had warned us not to and Dad and I got bad sunburns. My right foot got so badly burned my second toe turned purple for a long time. We used a lot of Noxema that week.

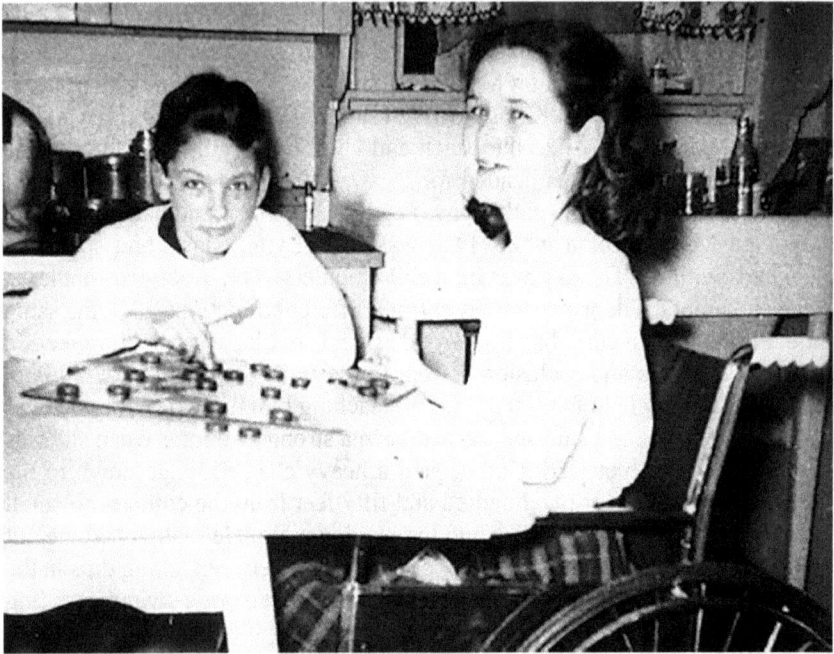

Checkers

We played a lot of Checkers and I got pretty good at beating Jackie. I was especially good at Chinese Checkers, but on Cape Cod that summer we played regular Checkers. Jackie didn't like to lose, so he would sometimes cheat to win. I got unbearably frustrated with his cheating and finally when I couldn't stand it any longer, I threw the checker board up in the air in a fury of anger and the checkers landed all over the room, on and under everything. I burst into tears, shouted "meaningless" things and didn't know what to do with myself. Jackie was stunned. Dad and Ma were shocked and Paul scurried outside, because none of them had ever seen me angry like that before. After that day, on the rare times I did get angry, I reached for anything nearby and threw it. Like the Checker Board. My anger came up fast and exploded, but it quickly turned inward into shame and fear and I would be overwhelmed with regret and humiliation. It was made worse this time because I loved Jackie. He was my friend. I felt horrible when I got mad. I wasn't ever supposed to and when I did it was just awful and I was so ashamed of such a major flaw in my character. Weakness when I was supposed to stay strong. The formula was, losing control—weakness. At all costs I must learn to keep control of my emotions and senses, because in my family, losing control was the most outrageous crime we could commit. Except for Ma. She was given grace in the matter. Ma would lose control with Peggy and scream a screeching tirade at the top of her lungs. Her rage would really boil over. She blamed Peggy for all and everything and directed every speck of her frustration and anger at her. Ma piled up all the anger in our family and hurled it at Peggy. I don't know if she ever showed Peggy any gentleness. She admired her beauty and popularity, but quickly related it to her own remembered youth. But she took her praise away as quickly as she offered it.

Ma didn't direct any of her screaming tirades at me, even if deep down it was me and my Polio she resented and felt guilty about. I felt the closeness of her anger and made sure I didn't ignite any of it. I tried to stay in control no matter what. It didn't matter that I was going to be thirteen that summer and on my first vacation since Island Falls. Only this vacation I was paralyzed and held hostage in my wheelchair–unable to walk in the sand or swim in the clear blue water–unable to do all the things I wanted to do in summer at the beach with Jackie and Paul. All I could do was watch and see, get hot all over, get sunburnt and never get to go in the water again. Especially that–never to go in the water again. Never to feel the waves in the ocean again. Never to feel the sand squish between my toes again and feel Jackie splash me playfully as I run on the beach. Never to walk into the waves again. Especially when I loved to do just that. And especially when I loved to stay in the water until I was blue and wrinkled. I grieved the loss of more than my childhood that summer. I grieved the loss of my silent control of things. I was now fully naked–exposed once and for all. My retreats into silence could from now on become suspect–my special hiding place given away–exposed and the only dumb thing that gave me away was my out-of-control rage, just because Jackie cheated at a stupid Checker game. Stop! Stop! Crash! Bang! Everyone stepped back in sudden surprise. And everyone turned away. And I turned away. It was too much rage and too much grief. Too much sadness. I had to pull myself together. Stop behaving like a spoiled kid. Stop making Jackie feel bad. Stop making Ma look at me like that. I had to stop feeling so ashamed of loosing control. Jackie picked up the Checker Board and set up all the pieces. Dad said, "It's okay, Stevie, it's okay." And Ma said it was a hot day and we were all a little tired.

I loved my little Paul more than anything. He was brown and soft and easy to be with. He was gentle and funny. He and Jackie went down to the beach where Jackie showed off for him. Showed him how strong he was. He tossed rocks into the water. And then the biggest show of all, he and Paul climbed up on a steep sand-dune, as a yellow Piper Cub airplane was flying over. Jackie (Superman) picked up a rock and looking up into the clear blue sky he said to Paul, "Watch this! I will hit that plane with this rock!" And sure enough. He heaved that rock into the air and Paul saw him do it! Jackie hit the wing of the Piper Cub Airplane with the rock! Just ask Paul! He'll tell you today, even as a man and a Catholic Priest, just exactly how Jackie threw that rock up into the sky and hit the wing of that plane. Jackie was Paul's Super Hero from then on and he held onto that moment of summer magic forever.

Years later as "knowing" adults Jackie and I were sitting together on the sun deck at North St in Stoneham and Jackie (then fifty-eight) confessed the truth about the airplane incident. He said "The plane happened to be flying unusually low–about a thousand feet–whizzing toward and by us and in that strangely synchronized moment, as I heaved the rock upward, the wing of the plane dipped and caught the flash of a sun ray on the tip of its wing and for a mini-moment the flash caused us to lose sight of the rock and it appeared to hit that very spot on the plane where the flash occurred. Of course," he said, "In a Jungian sense and in the boy's eye, that rock *did* hit that plane."

Jackie cautioned, "But we must not ever tell Paul, because that little miracle could have been that prime moment of spiritual insight that ultimately motivated him to join the Priesthood."

We shall not tell Paul, we agreed.

That summer at North Truro was the summer before Jackie and I went into the eighth grade–the last summer of our childhood, really, for both me and Jackie. After that, life got tougher and tougher. For me, because I had to manage so much control, I had to freeze up to do each day. I had to get smaller and smaller so I didn't hurt so much inside my barbed wire cage. In eighth grade, Jackie went on an academic strike in school, was not promoted and had a hard time getting over it. My life changed too after that summer and never was quite the same again.

Spinal Integrity

It was the next summer–1953. I started to cry and couldn't stop for days. I cried and cried and cried as my Birthday came and went and it turned to July again. I was re-admitted to Division 36 because it was decided that I likely would have surgery in order to correct the excessive curvature of my spine. The first thing I learned upon landing at Division 36 again was that since her marriage to Ken, Miss Wentworth was no longer working that unit. When it was finally decided that I would have the surgery, I was transferred to 5 Lower–the Orthopedic Surgical Unit. I had been in almost all of the private, semiprivate and multi-bed rooms on Division 36 whereas 5 Lower was much different. It was a Ward of twelve beds for girls in one wing and twelve beds for boys in the other wing, with a Nurses' station in the center. Each Ward had six beds against one wall and six beds against the other wall. But I wasn't there for more than a few days when I began to cry again. Because it didn't look like I was crying for any obvious reason no one asked Why? And no one stopped. Everyone kept moving. Even Miss McGinnis came through 5 lower and kept right on going. Dr. Grice walked by. No one stopped. I got the idea that I could cry as long as I wanted to until I was finished. Just as no one asked *why* words of comfort weren't offered either. "Let her work it out," they probably said. They must have thought that it would make me tough and strong, so I would be ready to tackle the life that was to come. Don't weaken her. Let her learn to be tough. Yes, that's what they must have said to themselves.

The obvious was not so obvious. I was alone and under the spell of immense grief, like none other I had ever experienced. I realized that I would never wear a party dress and walk in high heel shoes. Not ever. Uncontrollable tears–nonstop tears for days and days and days. The tears wouldn't/couldn't, didn't stop. The nurses and doctors–Miss McGinnis and Dr. Grice walked by my bed, looked at me, smiled and walked away. Strangely enough, Ma stopped and was the only one to stop. She sat very close to me, her face close to my face–listening, caring, wanting to understand. She said that I was probably unhappy because Division 36 was new and nice and 5 Lower was old and dilapidated. I figured some of the staff would likely be thinking that I was crying because I left Division 36 where Miss Wentworth had been and now I was in with all these new kids on 5 Lower. No. I cried because I wouldn't ever wear a party dress and walk in high heel shoes. Never. Not ever. I was grieving the loss of a way of life. The verdict was in. My time to grow and be alive was denied by the tribunal. I was alone and would remain alone in my metal cage for the rest of my entire lifetime and I was only fourteen.

I met Lena that summer. Our friendship lasted that whole year while we both were preparing for and recovering from our Spinal Fusions. Lena was twelve and our beds were side by side on 5 Lower. It was a summer of record breaking heat, plaster body casts, turn buckles, Doctor's Rounds, parent's getting to know each other, forbidden ice cream sodas, lots of laughter and lots of pain. On 5 Lower that summer we giggled, laughed, outwitted the doctors, made fun of the nurses and told stories about them. There were nurses we liked and nurses we didn't like. Some were all business and some joined in our fun and brought us the forbidden ice cream sodas. Some kids were really sick. Sandy, who was thirteen, had her leg amputated and Doctor Glimshire walked off the Ward with his arm around her mother's shoulder. "Doctor Glimshire. Doctor Melvin Glimshire." The Paging system called out his name over and over again and he would twirl around in a fury of swears to respond with the nearest phone. He was tall, with piercing dark eyes and rumpled dark brown hair. I liked him. He was loud and tough, but he was straight forward.

He was for real and knew how to feel. Unlike Doctor Mayo who was stiff and seemed to have no feelings at all. There was no interaction with him. He didn't know how to make contact with us. One day he had a hole in his white pants. He stood by my bed and Lena who happened to be nearby stuck her finger in the hole and startled him. He turned around quickly and stared at Lena with a shocked look on his face and Lena and I both laughed. Usually though, Lena was scared to death of the doctors. I watched her get more and more nervous as they made their rounds from bed to bed. By the time they got to Lena she would be crying uncontrollably. They'd talk to her and tease her until she laughed a little. Next they came to me. I wasn't scared. My crying was finally done and I just liked to be quiet and check them out. They were checking me out, so I was checking them out. As they ganged around my bed, I had their number. Doctor Banks would ask a question to which I usually knew the answer and I watched to see which doctor would volunteer an answer. Sometimes, if I liked the doctor who was on the receiving end of the question, I would say the answer and he would pick up on it and elaborate his response. Doctor Banks was wise to me. He would give me the eye and wink at me as he moved from my bedside to the next.

July and August had many days over 100 degrees on 5 Lower and several of us spent those days in plaster casts getting ready for the spinal fusions to straighten out the curvatures in our spines that each of us had acquired one way or another. My curvature was caused by Polio and the other kids had curvatures of different or unknown origin. Plaster of Paris jackets were wrapped all around our bodies, extending down one arm and down the opposite leg to just above the knee. One by one we had our turn in the Plaster Room where the casts were applied. I remember an elderly lady who worked in the Plaster Room rolling stockinet material. She was always suspicious that the doctors were whispering about her, because she was deaf and couldn't hear them. They seemed to enjoy teasing her and she seemed to enjoy the attention. The atmosphere in the Plaster Room was playful, although the work was really not playful. I spent a lot of time there. The Room was very hot and making plaster casts was hard work. I lay on a table with stockinet material covering my entire body, as rolls upon rolls of wet Plaster of Paris was wrapped down my left arm to my elbow and down the right leg to my knee. Before the plaster hardened, the body of the cast was carved out on both sides and a turn buckle was installed on one side. Over the next month my spine got straightened out by turning the turn buckle until my spine was straight inside the cast and held there. Three of us prepared for Spinal Fusions on 5 Lower that summer. In the night, the kids who could get up and walk came to our bedsides and helped us turn the buckles back and stuffed a bath towel in to relieve the pain. Lena got really scared one time. She over-slept and doctors making Rounds caught her before she had the turn buckle back in place.

I had my surgery on September 23rd. I don't remember the pain that followed, but I do remember the Morphine shots. How good I felt when the shot began to take effect. How I faded from reality and slid into unconsciousness. One day, Doctor Mayo was examining me and as he held my leg from which they had taken the bone to graft to my spine, my leg, which was in a plaster cast, slipped from his hand and landed with a thud on the bed. I cried out loud–cried way beyond the pain caused by drop-ping my leg. The crying was for all the small hurts when I didn't cry. I felt like a fake because I knew I cried too much for that one time. But it just felt good to cry and cry and cry and cry. So I did. Like a little kid who cries bigger than the hurt. Longer than the hurt–much longer than the hurt until someone said "knock it off!" And eventually I stopped. A Morphine shot finally stopped my tears that day.

Home in My Own Room

Back at home, after the Spinal Fusion, I was in the Plaster of Paris body cast for six months. While I was hospitalized, a new room had been added to our house for me, so I could have my own bedroom with my own bath-room and a door leading out to the backyard. The cost of the new room was $2,000.00 and Dad's friends at the electric Company held a raffle to help him pay for it. Dad painted the walls pink and Ma bought white curtains for the two windows. My bed was moved into the new room and Ma had her dining room back. She got an extra-long cord that reached my bed and every day for six months Lena and I talked on the phone. I began to manicure my nails then. Ma still took care of me–meals, baths and bedpan. She brushed my hair and saw to it I had something to read or the radio to listen to. Ma's friend, Wini Russel, gave me a Parakeet and I named him Teddy. He would fly around the room, land on my bed and walk all over my body cast. He would perch on my breakfast tray and dance around the edges of my grapefruit.

Paul was six in 1953 and he would hop into bed with me for a story or to watch TV. He kept my heart warm inside all that Plaster of Paris. Peggy was a Senior in High School that same year and basked in the glory she received for the lead role in *Father of the Bride*. Although Paul Murphy was her steady boyfriend by then, boys from the high school called for dates and lots of times Peggy had more boy friends than she knew what to do with. She wanted to be an Air Line Hostess.

Fern P. Heath was my Home Tutor who came from the Stoneham School System. Earlier, in June of that year, Saint Patrick's Grammar School gave me my Eighth Grade Diploma. Mrs. Heath did the best she could to keep me up to date on my lessons and would come for one hour three days a week. By then my classmates were in Ninth Grade and I was getting what Mrs. Heath could give me of English, History and Math. Mostly she gave me of herself. And now, many years later, I remember her love of words and nature–her love for Leslie, her husband and her daughters, Hazel and Ginger, who were adults then with families of their own. Mrs. Heath got excited when the grass turned green in Spring time. When I graduated from High School Mrs. Heath gave me a copy of *The Brothers Karamazov* and inside the cover she inscribed the following words: "To Barbara, who has so much to give. Always invest your energy wisely in those things that will most enrich your life."

In the morning I woke up about eight a.m. turned on the radio beside the bed and listened to Allan Derry with his disc jockey talk, Eddie Fisher singing *Oh My Papa* and Pattie Page singing *How Much Is That Doggie In The Window*. Ma cranked up my bed and set the breakfast tray in front of me. After I used the bed pan, she brought a basin of warm water so I could wash up. Then it was time for me to get up and Ma put on my body jacket, called a Bivalve because it was split down the front and could be sprung apart to slide into. It was made of plastic with three straps across the front to hold it secure. I wore it whenever I sat up to keep my spine straight and to support the diaphragm. I couldn't breathe easily without my diaphragm being supported and my scoliosis was progressing. The morning was exercise time and Mrs. Elliott would come over to give Ma some help. At the Polio Clinic Ma had been shown how to do it and we were sent back home with the expectation that Doctor's Orders would be followed. And, indeed, they became like the dictates of The Church. The black metal leg braces had brown leather straps that stretched across my knees and thighs and were attached to the brown leather oxfords. Leather and elastic straps connected the braces to the bottom of my body jacket and those straps became substitutes for muscles.

Ma put all that equipment on me while I was still in bed. Then Mrs. Elliott helped her stand me up against the living room wall, where before Polio I used to sit beside the big console radio and listen to "The Green Hornet." The two of them would get on either side of the chair, lift me up to a standing position, then they would put the Canadian Crutches around my arms and in my hands to give me the support I needed to stand there and balance myself for about fifteen minutes, or until I was too tired to stand any longer. Then they would sit me back down in the wheelchair again, where I'd wait for Mrs. Heath to come for my school lessons.

Eventually the standing exercise progressed to a walking exercise. Ma helped me up beside the bed where I stood until I caught my balance and felt okay. Then I would work my way across the room to the opposite wall where the full length mirror hung. I watched myself as I moved to make sure I was keeping my shoulders and body straight. The right crutch, the left leg, the left crutch, the right leg. Carefully, thoughtfully, keeping my balance and watching the mirror. Swing to my right and my left foot cleared the floor. Swing to my left and my right leg cleared the floor. It took about ten minutes to cross ten feet, to the mirror. Then I turned around and rested against the wall, before heading back across the room. The exercise took every ounce of my energy. It was a prescribed discipline, religiously carried out every

119

morning, Monday through Fri-day. One day at the Polio Clinic in Doctor Grice's presence, Miss Volland, my Physical Therapist, expressed the obvious reality that walking was probably not going to be a useful way for me to move about in the world. Doctor Grice did not appreciate the starkness of her comment. He looked at me and said "We can dream, can't we?" And that was its essential usefulness–the ultimate dream goal of my physical rehabilitation. To walk again, even if it was only across a small room. Yes, walking was the goal of all the exercises, all the surgeries, all the Thursday mornings at the Polio Clinic. Walking was the goal that once reached, could release me from paralysis and direct me toward getting on with my life in a wheelchair.

"We bear in our bodies
the dying of Christ
so that His life
may be become
manifest in us."

YELLOW

VIBRANT YELLOW

VELVET YELLOW LARGE AND DEEP

AND ALIVE

WITH EXCITEMENT YELLOW YELLOW YELLOW

I HAVE BEEN YELLOW

FOR A LONG TIME NOW

YELLOW LIKE A PANSEY

IN SUMMER

WITH A DEEP PURPLE CENTER

THE YELLOW PANSEY

THAT APPEARS ALONG A BORDER

OR IN A WINDOW BOX

QUIET AND STILL

FULL AND RICH AND ALIVE

IN THE MIDDLE OF THINGS

VISIBLE AND CLEAR AND DISTINCT

YELLOW YELLOW YELLOW

WALLS OF YELLOW

A YELLOW SWEATER

ALWAYS YELLOW

DEEP-RICH-VELVETY-

YELLOW

STILL

QUIET

ALIVE

IN THE MIDST OF THINGS

YELLOW

I arise this morning
to remember
and give praise and thanks.
to the everlasting beauty
that is in me.
That same beauty that is in you.
that beauty that I see in you
that reflects back to me
all of who I am. I see me in you.
I see my wholeness
my strength and gentle beauty.
I see in you
the fragments of my life the broken, fragile pieces
of my very self-Broken
Yes I see me in you.
And all of me drops to my knees
in humble recognition
of myself.
I am in awe of myself.
I see me in you.
All of me. A piece here.
Another piece there until I am whole again.
And I rise from my knees -
I stand very straight
and tall and strong.
I inhale deeply
and I exhale just as deeply
The all of me alive and
Everlasting.

Memory Can Be Ever So Deceiving

I don't know if I really could balance my wheelchair on the back wheels and bounce down the single step from the front hall to the porch at the house on Cottage Street, or not. In my memory I think I did that. I can almost feel the rush of holding my balance and the grounding of my chair as I landed strongly and safely. But I know I couldn't have got myself back in. To bring the small front wheels up over the step and then lean foreword enough to swing the rest of the chair and myself over that doorstep. No, I'm sure I didn't do that. And somewhere in my memory I have the sensation of bouncing down a flight of stairs, too. The same way I remember going down that one step. And I'm almost pretty darned sure I never did that. I have confusion–ambivalence in my memory around what was real for me and what I thought about and wished was real. I do know this for sure. In our house on Cottage Street I used my manual chair without the sides on and I felt safe–not afraid of loosing my balance. I became accustomed to life lived in my wheelchair, developing a casualness, as I sat on one foot tucked under my other leg, Or I used my good arm and hand and managed to get my legs crossed Indian style. I see the modern day version of myself now in the way the young newbies to paralysis use their sports chairs and participate in the fullness of athletics and life. So much has changed and not changed.

The years between 1950 and 1963 from when I was ten, then a teenager and then in my early twenties. They were the infantile paralysis years. I struggled against the paralysis of my body as hard as I struggled against the paralysis of my family. We were all paralyzed. My polio simply reflected and manifested the paralysis of the total family. We couldn't get beyond the devastating sickness of our paralysis. I was forever the sick child. The *victim* of polio. The *invalid*. Yes in-valid, you see? *Not valid!* There was no one to notice that we were broken and I was missing my validity. If only we, or I could call out and say "Look! See it! This is what is going on here!" And so we all struggled along in ugly loneliness and isolation, unnoticed by loving eyes and minds.

There was so much empty time. Lonely time. Boring time. Eventually, I learned to knit and paint and do embroidery. All to pass the time. To have something to do. To fill up empty space. To keep busy. I sat in the living room in the evenings and thought that God must want me to be doing this right now or else he'd show me the way to do something else. He must want me to be right here, right now, doing exactly what I'm doing. Because I thought and thought and thought and there was no other way for me to be doing anything else right now, other than what I was doing.

Years later, I talked with Jackie about those years and he said it sounded like a kind of Zen thing. I thought that may have been partially true, but I couldn't see Zen jelling with such intense loneliness. Basically, I turned my thoughts off during those years. I knitted sweaters and scarves and mittens, did crewel embroidery and made ornaments for Christmas. I hoped that someone who could lead me out of this lonely place would come along, but no one came.

Reading began to nudge, then lift me up out and away from despair. I dived into Thomas Merton's books: *Seven Story Mountain, Waters of Siloe, No Man Is An Island*–all of them. I loved them. When I read Merton I was not confined in time or space. I was free. My mind united with all the minds everywhere. Especially the minds and hearts of people who were far away in other parts of the world. My consciousness merged with their consciousness. I felt connected. It became a whole other reality. I was transported to a world more real than the physical world that kept me anchored in that isolated, lonely place. This new reality had no boundaries, no limits. I felt alive and finally connected–connected to energy as far away as South America, China, Russia and Europe. Wherever my thoughts took me, I would go. I would hold a Merton book in my hands and read a few lines, or a page and be so far away from where I sat. Deep, deep down inside of myself and far away from where I actually was. Merton fed my mind, my soul, my heart and my imagination. It was hard to be confined then. In my mind, I began to resist always being at home with Ma and Dad. I wanted to be out there, somewhere, with friends. I was small and tight and confined. Dad took me out for a ride on Saturday afternoons. We'd ride to Georgetown or West Newbury along the Merrimac River. We wouldn't talk. We'd just ride and I'd have imaginary conversations with imaginary people. I created an entire imaginary life. People and places and things to do. I took pride in that imaginary world, like it was more real than real and it was lots better. It was superior. I felt okay there. I had something to hold on to there. I was okay there. Even now when I'm scared and when I feel overwhelmed and inferior and unable to keep up, I escape into my imaginary world. It's still there for me. I go there and take comfort in those old familiar friends and familiar sur-roundings. It is totally my world–a world that only I know about and only I can go there. For me, it's real and it's safe. I can make it be any way I want it to be. And I can make me be any way I want me to be.

> "It's a lovely reality
> when someone's dream
> is
> loved into Being"

Dreams and Barbed Wire Cages

When was it I dared to dream? When did I catch a glimpse of freedom from my barbed wire prison? Yes, I remember when I dared to dream. When I dared to catch a glimpse–a glimpse quickly smothered and put away. Yes, I remember a time when I dared to dream. A time of anger. A time of deep, dark and burning rage–when I lost control and shouted meaningless words– meaningless words hot with anger and streaming tears–steaming, streaming red hot tears and meaningless words. RAGE! When I lost control. When I threw to the floor whatever I had in my hand. Lost my temper and wanted with all my strength and beyond all my strength to run away–to get away as far away as I could. Oh yes, I remember a time when I dared to dream. When I felt so overwhelmed by it all that I dared to dream of escaping to freedom– running away out of it all, until I exhausted all of my strength and fell back into a place of dark despair. A hollowed-out-ness with no hope of escape–a bottomless decent into emptiness. The gaping emptiness of loss, where there was no one, no other one to hear my despair–the over whelming weakness, the utter powerlessness and loss of control of Infantile Paralysis and deep shame and humiliation. The only voices around me were ridiculing, criticizing ones, because I lost control. "How unlike YOU!" they would say. It was in the emerging shadow of those discomforting words that I dared (learned) to dream of escaping to freedom.

When I was twelve and Peggy was fifteen she created a scene and I wanted to explode from my chair. Instead I had a glass Christmas ornament in my hand and I threw it with all my might toward her and it crashed to the floor in pieces. Ma yelled "Stop!" "Stop!" And I shouted out mountains of those meaningless words!

Humiliation. Shame. Nowhere to hide. No way to run and hide. And when I was older, there were other rare times, rare moments when all of my anger and rage and frustration burst out of control and I felt so deeply ashamed defeated exposed and vulnerable. I vowed never, never, ever again to show my soul so plainly before them. They had no idea what was going on with me–of my dream to escape–to get away from THEM–to go away and NEVER come back. Had Polio not burst into my life and taken charge, by God, I would have gone to California with Jackie in 1960, when he was twenty and I was twenty. I would have poured all of myself on the streets of San Francisco. Yes, I would have done that! Let it all go. All of that hot burning consuming rage, sadness and disappointment... gone!

Yes, I do remember a time when I dared to dream. Dared to dream of escape–leaving them–Ma and Dad, until my strength was sapped and I was withered from frustration and hopelessness and reason with all its matter-of-factness, would come back in to remind me, how could I escape? How could I? When I couldn't take care of myself–when my whole world was kept from me? When the easiest thing for others was to do for me, rather than have me do for myself. I was less of a burden when I complied and let others do it for me. It was easier if I just remained passive (detached) and let them have their way. Yes, let them do it all. *Reason*, with all its matter-of-factness, drained me of all my energy, passion, and hope–*all of it*! I was left empty–hollowed out of all my dreams–the dreams that had flashed momentarily out of my rage–squelched before they had a chance to become even a possibility. And still, here now, even at age fifty-two I continue to squelch the dream. I medicate my hot burning stomach ulcer pains and wait. Wait for my time to escape–to be free of them.

"RETURN

OH MY SOUL

TO YOUR TRANQUILITY.

FOR GOD HAS BEEN GOOD TO YOU.

HE HAS FREED MY EYES FROM TEARS,

MY FEET FROM STUMBLING.

MY SOUL FROM DEATH.

I WILL WALK BEFORE GOD

IN THE LAND OF THE LIVING."

Psalm 116:9

When, where did I find that psalm to repress dreaming even more? Piety and reason conspiring together. Am I solely in this world to give others the opportunity to serve? Is it my place to provide for others an exercise in charity? To give others an opportunity to be of service?

127

Paul said: "Give Peggy a chance to be kind to you. If she wants the house, give it to her! She'll let you live there. Let her be kind to you." For fifty-two fucking years I gave Ma that chance to be kind to me. And earning her salvation that way, she damn near killed me with kindness.

NO! NO! NO! Is it then, for me to learn humility and let go of my dreams? My fragmented, undeveloped dreams? My dreams born of rage and frustration when Ma would say, "You're too skinny. No one will love you. You can't cook. No one will love you. You would be too much of a burden for him. Never want anything and you'll never be disappointed." Assuring for herself a companion to be at her side all the days of her life! When was it that I dared to dream?

When is it now that I dare to dream? I stay inside this barbed wire. So still. Even at age fifty-two, until rage comes along again to frighten me again–to scare me stiff. When Peggy says, "Why haven't you moved out! Mother would be better off without you! This is my mother and father's home! My brother's home! You just live here!"

If I stay crouched down, silent inside the barbed wire. If I just stay perfectly still, it won't hurt so much. I won't hurt so much. I'll just stay still–frozen–inert... Infantile–Paralysis.

SO I BECOME FOR OTHERS THE ONE WHO COMES ALONG AND SAYS, "YES, YOU CAN!" Not only yes you can, but, YES, YOU MUST! You must dream your dreams and create ways to make them come true. YOU MUST! YOU MUST! You have to and I'll help you. I'll cheer you on. I'll become for you what I needed to be for me. I'll help you create your dreams. I'll help you not be afraid of your dreams. I'll think with you of ways to make your dreams come true.

First of all, DREAM! "What do you want for you?" Dare to dream. And I will take you by the hand and you will see there is a way to make your dream come true.

Was there no one there for me? Was there no one there to say "Dream." No. Of course not! Because others were there to quickly say, "DO IT THIS WAY." Do it that way. I know what's best for you." If you do what I say. If you do what I want you to do. If you'll do it *my* way, I'll support your plan. Otherwise you're on your own kid and you'll fail because you can't make it without me."

Inside my barbed wire prison I am on my own. I still dream fragments of my dream. I take bits and pieces of my dreaming and I cling to mythical figures. I find my way inside the barbed wire. My dreams burst forth from deep inside of me. Like an erupting volcano. The hot burn-ing lava emerges from an inner world unseen and unheard of, unknown, even to myself. In all of the mystery of our planet earth, the inside of the earth and the inside of me. Where dreams are. Where dreams burst forth. Frightening. Scary. Too frightening. I remember when I dared to dream...

But I am learning, aren't I

"It's a lovely reality

when

someone's dream

is

loved into being."

I try so hard to trace its origin. When did I begin to weave my barbed wire cage? Was that before Polio? When did I realize I needed to say "no" to the life urge inside of me? When did I shrivel up and start to die inside? Did I do it right away? Before Polio? Did I do that when I failed to thrive as an infant–when I stopped eating as an infant? Did I decide early on that I did not like this lifetime very much–did I pull back right then and there from the source of life here on earth? Did I begin way back then to watch and to see and to stay very still? Did I begin even then (before Polio) to weave a tight cage of barbed wire around me to keep people out and to keep me in?

Ma and Dad had stopped dreaming too. Dad stopped dreaming when his dog, Pep, was killed on the first day he had him. The child pain inside him stayed raw within him his whole life. I knew how sad he was about it because when Peggy and I would ask him for a puppy he would say, "No, no dogs." And then one day he told us about "Pep" and the way he told us, I knew how sad he was about it, so I stopped asking for one.

And Ma created her barbed wire protection on Christmas day when she was three and there was no Christmas dinner–no celebration, as the lady and mother of the house lay dead drunk on the kitchen floor. So Ma created her own protection from it all and married a man who became part of her own barbed wire protection. So there they were posing as adults–teetotalers– abstaining from alcohol and abstaining from emotions that might cause any sort of residual pain–any pain–abstaining from intimacy and closeness–abstinence from dreaming. Separate lives locked in pain–not knowing–just not knowing–abstaining from alcohol, life and the nourishment of love.

Dying the way a dedicated alcoholic dies, depleted, worn out, devoid of warm human touches–locked in behind the barbed wire, living each day mechanically–adult children, willing to follow all the rules made by someone else. Tight rules. Clearly defined rules. Catholic rules. Working class rules. Government rules, like the one printed in front of the Post Office, "KEEP OFF THE GRASS." And that grass was so inviting. The great tacit rule–Live by the rules blindly and you will be safe from dreaming. Obedience becomes the highest good. Obey God's rules. Don't think. Don't feel. Don't dream. Obey God's authority on earth. Stay tight. Don't stray. Keep the Faith. Fight the Good Fight. Stay tight inside the barbed wire cage of martyrdom–of Sainthood–of obedience! Obey all the rules and you'll get through this lifetime DEAD, finished, finished off!!! Ma's lifelong advice to me: "Never want anything and you'll never be disappointed."

Still, when was it that I dared to dream? Was it in the Iron Lung? Was it when I broke open and lost control, screaming against the alienation, isolation hurt and pain? When precisely was it I could take no more, so I screamed, threw things, then quickly retreated behind the barbed wire again–retreated when I saw myself respond in Peggy's way and I knew the screeching tirade that would follow. When? When? When was it that I dared to dream? A flash? A moment? The guilt, the anxiety, the fear–the flaming pain in my gut that radiated under my arms across my back throughout my chest and around my heart–until I screamed and screamed and screamed in silence and pulled back tight and small and safe behind the barbed wire again and again–way down inside where no one could come in and where I can't get out. When did I dare to dream? Did it emerge from inside the books, in words–silent, secret words? Words like: "Man's capacities have never been measured..." or "Every man is new in nature..." Liberating words... "In the beginning was the word" ...the *word*.

Was it when I wept for three days and three nights when I was fourteen– when I was transferred from Division 36 to 5 Lower. When I had no words to say–heard no words and felt no words–just tears–tears of aloneness–no one to say what the tears were saying–only those who looked in, saw the tears and stayed away until the tears left. Three days and three nights to tame the wildness–the urge to have a life–to dream–three days and three nights to burn myself out–to wear myself out–to drain myself dry–to weep all the tears out of my fourteen-year-old paralyzed body. Give in! Give up! Obey! Go dead. Go dead inside. Dry up. Go passive. *Play dead so we don't have to deal with you.* Stay hidden. Don't let me see or have to deal with your feelings. Don't call on me. Don't call on me for emotional support because I refuse to recognize what you are feeling. Do not call on me. I don't deal with that part of you. The rule is this: If you want emotional support keep the hell away. Because if you don't you know the response you'll get if you do. So don't!

So, when did I dare to dream? On Christmas morning in 1950 when I sat up in my wheelchair for the first time? On Christmas when Paul and Peggy came to me in the hospital for the first time since July 20th when I was taken there? I dreamed of being able to push myself around in the wheelchair. I dreamed: If only I could... touch my chin, my tongue. Yes, I had dreamed the dream before, early on, when I dreamed, "if only I could..." rub my eyes, feed myself, use my one good hand. "If only I could..." then I'd never want any other thing again. "If only I could..." That dream (if only I could) repeated itself over like Gene Autry's song, *over and over and over and over again*. If only I could do just a little bit more than this, a little more, and a little more and a little more. Until I could do it all again. That lasted until I was sixteen, when I finally realized that I'd never do it all again, or even a small part of it all. Reality broke into my dreaming then and made dreaming so painful I put dreaming away. I blocked dreaming. I became deliberate: rational and PRACTICAL by any and all means. A new step by step progression toward something. Baby steps. I blocked dreaming then. I blocked feeling then. I froze my mind. I froze my heart too. I became mechanical and deliberate, unfeeling, no nonsense, step-by-step problem solving. Then I said "I must..." and "I have to..." and I became determined and deliberate.

All of me on the inside tightened. My smile remained on the outside, hollow and unauthentic, unreal. So the people I needed would stay around. Their rules, not mine. "Keep smiling!"

Who was I? What was I? How could I be in the world, isolated and alone like this, Deposited here to tough it out. Trapped. with no escape. No way out.

Oh... I remember those summer days of being alone–in my room–in the yard–unable to move independently. Entertained by what others brought to me. I did jigsaw puzzles and read whatever magazines and articles someone else brought to me that didn't particularly interest me. School friends by now were on their own way and a new girlfriend didn't come by–only rarely then did they come by. Even Jackie wasn't coming during the week as much because he was so into football, baseball and a new girlfriend, Linda Clark, who lived way down by the Melrose line and occupied by all the other stuff in Junior High School. There was no way out. There was no way out. Day after day after day and no one came and said "This way out." "Over here!"

"This way out!" My throat froze. My brain froze. All of me froze. And as I froze, Ma and Dad froze even more. Mechanical, deliberate, matter-of-fact, day after day after day.

131

So dreaming stopped... I was fourteen, then fifteen and becoming totally deliberate. I HAD TO GET OUT. I HAD TO TAKE ONE STEP AT A TIME AND GET THE FUCK OUT!!! In the total darkness—deliberate and determined. Every step required someone else's agreement. Someone had to agree and give permission. And then someone else had to make it happen. All of my life was dependent upon the agreement of someone else. "Please may I take one giant step?" So I played "Simon says." Sometimes Simon says "You may not." and sometimes Simon says "You may." Instead of dreaming I played "Simon Says." And my dreams and my feelings got buried alive again. They got pushed all the way back into my being. And I became short sighted. Near sighted, Step-by-step. I had to get out of this cage. Somehow. I had to get out. No one to talk to. No one to say "Follow me. I'll show you how. Come this way."

What happens to dreams deferred? Where do dreams go when we wake up?

The Girl of Yesterday & Today

I see all the shades of green in the grass today. The grass is yellow, blue, gray and brown. I thought the grass was only green until I sat here long enough to know it wasn't. I am here every day. On cool days in early spring and on the very hot days of mid July. And I am still here as the days get shorter and cooler in early Fall. My favorite spot is a small knoll–a tiny rise in the backyard that tilts my wheelchair just enough to compensate for my body being not entirely even and I need to lean to my left to catch my balance. The apple tree stands just behind me, over my left shoulder. It was the perfect size for a little girl to climb and stay up there for as long as she wanted. That was my spot then, as this is my spot now. I used to sit in the apple tree where the lower branches met and formed a natural seat. And I would be whomever I wanted to be– mostly a strong and free me. There was then and there is now something very deep down in me that I really like being. I'd rather be me than anyone else in the whole world. Sometimes I think that me is hiding Way down deep inside, crouching–just being–somewhere inside.

I especially liked me when I was perched in the apple tree, or like now, sitting here alone on my knoll, being the girl I am.

The girl I am today sees the different colors of the grass. And sees all the trees that are planted on our lawn and on Mrs. Elliott's lawn. The Blue Spruce is Mrs. Elliott's favorite–a medium size tree on the front lawn. It looks so fine–so perfectly symmetrical from top to bottom–so proud and full. Across the street is the Nagle's house with the tall Pine next to it. It's a very old house and not kept up very well. All the neighbors felt bad for the Nagles because Mrs. Nagle died and her daughter Deanie found her dead at the kitchen table. There were four daughters. Dot was the oldest and had the distinctive reputation of being a lady. She was tall and thin and had a job. But I liked Alice the best. She was friendly, smiled easily and would stop and talk with me. Ann was the youngest and was two years older than me. We use to play together, but not much since the polio. Ann did okay. She eventually got married and everyone was glad that she grew up with the fewest emotional scars.

Their father, Johnny Nagle, was a nice man. Ma used to say, "If there was a cloud in the sky, Johnny Nagel wouldn't go to work." The kids in the neighborhood loved him. He would pick blackberries with them and in winter sled with them on the slope beside his house–the kind of neighbor you don't see so much anymore. Not long after Mrs. Nagle passed on, Johnny Nagle had a heart attack and also died at home. Alice stayed in the house along with her husband, Shawn. Shawn worked for the Post Office and they had two children, Sandy and Michael. Mrs. Elliot and Ma used to worry about those kids, because they would run around the neighborhood with no clothes on, but they didn't seem to notice how happy the kids looked.

From my place here in the tiny knoll I can think and reflect about all of the neighbors who were around then–the Gustaferros, The Elliotts, the Nagles, the Vierras, the Gallellas. All good neighbors–people who, for the most part, minded their own business and thankfully like Ma said "didn't have many arguments over the kids." Mainly because the grownups let the kids settle most of their own problems and that worked out pretty well. They all remained there, each in their own space and each one caring in their own way about the others.

The Gustaferros lived on the other side of Mrs. Elliott. Mr. Gustaferro was a barber and had a garden. He and Dad liked to visit each other and discuss their gardens in the summertime. Mrs. Gustaferro (Anna) worked at the shoe factory. Her daughter Lena was twelve when Carl Junior was born. Ma took care of Junior while Mrs. Gustaferro worked.

Lena and Junior were especially smart and later when Paul and Junior were good friends, Junior taught Paul about Astronomy. They both had telescopes and would get all excited about the meteor showers.

Lena and Junior were expected to get all A's at school and mostly they did! Their house was immaculate! No one was allowed to wear shoes in their house! And their kitchen had mirrors all around. Ma couldn't believe how Mrs. Gustaferro kept those mirrors so shiny, but she surely did.

The biggest scandal that ever happened in our neighborhood happened to Lena. Two days before her wedding, her husband to be got arrested for the armed robbery of several gas stations! Mr. Gustaferro returned all the wedding presents.

The Gallellas lived next door to us on the south side. They owned the Twin Restaurant in the Square and they named it The Twin Restaurant because they had twins! Rita and James! The twins were one year older than Peggy and their other son, Joey, was one year older than Paul! Mr. Hastings was Mrs. Gallella's father and we especially liked him because he reminded us of Grampa. Mr. Hastings was Irish and liked to go into City Point in South

Boston to visit his cronies. Paul was very fond of Mr. Hastings. They sat together on Gallella's front steps and talked. Paul went to Mr. Hastings wake at Cassidy's Funeral Home and he was surprised that Mr. Hastings had on his best suit! He expected him to have pajamas on.

The Vierras lived across the street from the Gallellas, next to the Nagles. They owned a Variety Store in Cambridge and Mr. and Mrs. Vierra were gone all day every day. Danny, Lucy, Beadie and Jacky took care of each other. Sometimes Mrs. Vierra's sister, Franny, took care of them, too. Beadie and Peggy were good friends as were Paul and Jacky. I was in between. Danny and Lucy were older than the rest of us. The worst thing that ever happened to the Vierras was the time Mrs. Vierra ran over their dog Mister and killed him! That was awful and it upset Dad a lot.

Kate Corcoran lived two doors down on the other side of the Gallella's. Miss Corcoran was a School Teacher and never married. Ma called Miss Corcoran Kate! Kate took a lot of punishment from the neighborhood kids because she was constantly yelling at them to get out of the street and not ride their bikes on the sidewalk. She would call the cops on the big kids when they'd play baseball in the street and hit her house with a foul ball. Because of that, the kids hated Kate and did mean things to aggravate her. They threw eggs at her front door from behind the Vierra's hedges! One morning when Paul was about twelve, Kate came to our door with her hands full of apples! She told Ma that they were OUR apples and that Paul had thrown them into her Yard! Ma was soooo em-barrassed! She apologized and took the apples. Later, when Paul came home with Dad, she realized that he hadn't been home all morning, so Ma took the apples back to Kate's house and told her not only were they not OUR apples, but Paul had been at the lake with his Dad and was not even HOME when the incident occurred.

Another time, Paul and a few of his friends were throwing rotten apples at passing cars on Cottage Street. They thought they were only throwing at vehicles driven by people they didn't know, but one apple hit a car driven by Mr. Bishop, who lived just a few minutes away on Victoria Lane and knew Mrs. Duffy and Paul, who was caught red handed at the scene of the crime with a rotten apple still in his hand. Ma went wild on Paul that day!

Yes, there were many shades of green in the grass in our back yard. I liked to sit there and contemplate the variation of colors and think about the lives of all the people in our neighborhood. I liked it even better when someone came along and called me out of my aloneness.

Jesus wept

as he entered

Jerusalem

saying

"if they only knew..."

Take me to the center of myself, Lord. Take me by the hand and lead me deep within my soul. Take me there so I can see clearly again, simply and uncluttered. I didn't want to be there earlier. I wanted to be anywhere else. But now I want to be there. Because you granted my wish to be elsewhere, I have been elsewhere and I have had fun and have laughed and been in love and I have felt alive in this world. I want all of that to continue and I also want to go back to the quiet places you found for me so long ago. Bring me there, Lord.

To anchor myself to a different tone for the moment, what I really want to express here is how deeply I cherish my life, which I consider to be a gift from God and how important God is to me. I don't want to hide that from view. God was hard to find way back then when I prayed to believe in belief– to go back a step before believing. To believe in believing would have been enough. All of the God stuff was remote and reserved for churches and other religious stuff. I rejected all of that very early on and rejected the idea of God along with it. God was linked to the church and the church didn't appeal to me at all. I found a God-life inside of me in the back yard, looking at the grass. When I first saw the individual blades of grass and saw all the different colors that green is–all the shadows cast upon the grass–the short grass, the deep grass, the withered grass, the lush deep green grass, I saw me and I saw God in all the shades of green grass.

Yes, I found God-life within me and all around me in bed at night when my sadness and tears would surge up and wash my face with abundance. I felt God-life then all around me, beside me, above me, at the foot of my bed and inside of me. Lifting me up from my heaviness on the bed, supporting me completely. I could never quite make it all the way to despair because of that enduring presence of the God-life which enlivened me and said "keep going, you're okay, don't quit!"

Jesus wept

as he entered

Jerusalem

Saying

"If they only knew…"

Yahweh, my God, is the core of my being where everything makes sense. I retreat there. He has taught me how to get there. He sat me down many years ago and taught me how to find my way there. It took a long time, but he stayed with me. He stayed through hard times and he stayed through easy times. He stayed when I paid attention and he stayed when I didn't. God-life stayed in me all along. Even when I consciously separated myself from him, made myself "long gone." "Come back to me," he said, "Come back to the center of your self. This is how you get there. You sit very still for hours and hours and hours, for days and months and years. Yes. I mean that! I want you to be still. And listen. Deep inside of you. I want you to see all the shades of green there in your back yard–in the grass. And I want you to look up, way, way up into the deep blue sky. I want you to see all those puffy white clouds. See them move across the sky and hide behind Nagle's big, tall pine tree. See them dissipate altogether and be no more. Watch. Notice. See all there is to see in your backyard. Feel the absence of the sun's warmth on a cool, cloudy day, the chill and the grayness. And feel the sun's warmth and see its sparkling beauty on a sunny day when it shines on separate blades of grass, and sparkles. Watch how the sun settles now and then on a flower, a zinnia, an aster, a purple aster. Just sit there in your backyard in May, in June, in July, in August for hours at a time, without a book to read, without a friend to be there with you. Just you, sitting in your wheelchair–looking around, looking deeply into the grass. Perched on the uneven knoll. Tilted a little. Chilled sometimes. Too warm other times.

I know you weep. I know you cry. I know you don't want to be here. I know. And I weep, too. Find me there. Take this time. It's okay and you know it's okay. Be patient. The hurt and the pain and the darkness will all go away someday. It is important for you to find your way in and out of your soul." Listen. Listen to the sound of no sound.

137

Lennie

I was fifteen in 1954 and after endless summer days. I needed to go to school!

My routine was broken by visits to the Polio Clinic every six weeks. Doctor Grice took my left hand in both of his strong hands and talked ahead about surgery that would transplant muscles and graft from bone and eventually could re-create a functional hand for me. Miss McGinnis, my ever present Social Worker, thought ahead to Boston University and said, "Down the road I'll introduce you to that world and Alice Gambel." I was angry with her then because I wanted to go to High School NOW! My need was immediate. I wanted something, now! I thought Miss McGinnis was missing the point of my whole existence. Her solutions were for a future time, another world, distant and remote when I needed answers "right now." but every time I mentioned school to her, Miss McGinnis would repeat, "Yes, I'll introduce you to Alice Gambel at Boston University when you're ready." AGGGGHHHHHH!

Mrs. Heath still came to the house for one hour for my tutoring each day but by then we were accomplishing very little academically. But more importantly, she was the thread that kept me connected to the outside world where kids my age were going to school. I was ready. I wanted and needed to move beyond my bedroom–beyond physical therapy–beyond surgeries– beyond the backyard in Summertime. I wanted and needed to get on with my life and no one knew how to direct me then in 1954 when I was fifteen. Ma and Dad had all they could do to keep going day after day.

But there was Bill MacKay who came into our life. He was Chairman of the local March of Dimes and befriended Ma and Dad shortly after I was *stricken*. A Polio *Victim* himself Bill was a big man with an obvious limp in his gait. He was a powerful friend to the *stricken* families. *Stricken*. That was the familiar language used to describe people and families who had Polio. *Stricken*. *Victim*. Now we refer to ourselves not as *victims*, but as *survivors*. Not as *stricken*, but as *challenged*. Bill had town political connections and worked hard to raise money that paid for my treatments. Ma and Dad were grateful for his help and friendship. Bill and Dad shared their love of fishing and became good personal friends. Ma especially liked his wife Elsie. She was stylish and smart. Elsie's white hair was piled high on her head and her blue eyes blinked repeatedly when she spoke with animated enthusiasm about education and the hope she saw in young people. Elsie and Bill took personal pride in my slow, tiny gains in strength and function. Bill didn't stop his tears from streaming down his cheeks the day he watched me walk a few feet from the side of my bed to the wall. All his hard work for The March of Dimes paid off in that moment. And Bill dreamed his dreams for me, "Someday maybe you will open a card shop." Another time he dreamed out loud, "Perhaps you will have an answering service." I had heard all of them so I smiled my *sweet little polio girl* smile. I watched Elsie. She was a teacher. She was a School Committee Member. I knew I didn't want a card shop or an answering service. Not big enough or important enough for *Me*.

If it weren't for Bill and Elsie, I never would have met Lennie–their adopted son. Lennie became my good friend when I was fourteen, fifteen and sixteen and Lennie was eighteen, nineteen and twenty. Lennie hated high school, but when I was getting to know him he was back to school for post-graduate classes. He frequently skipped his classes and came over to see me.

Big Lennie. Big talkin' Lennie, full of expansive feelings and good humor. He was about 5'10" and real stocky at well over 200 lbs. He had brown hair cut in a crew cut which made his full face seem fat. His deep brown, penetrating eyes saw everything. He always needed a shave and his full lips revealed strong, white teeth when he smiled, which he did a lot. Lennie's smile told lots of stories. His smiles were wise, sarcastic, warm, and funny. "He's a bum," Dad said. And Lennie would always leave before Dad got home at quarter to five. "A pain in the neck," Ma called him, even though she liked him. She would engage in friendly banter and lightly flirt with him. Then after a while, barely tolerated him. That was Ma's way with men–friendly, flattering, teasing at first. Then cool, detached and distant. She would leave us and get on with her housework. Lennie was good entertainment–great company for me. And he was Elsie's boy and Ma liked Elsie. So even when she didn't want Lennie around, she kept quiet about it because she didn't want to offend Elsie. Lucky for me, Lennie was not only a good gregarious all around guy but he also brought a whole new window of the world to me. He loved Art, Music and Literature. He would go to the Library and bring back a book or a record or an art reproduction. He loved Judy Collins and we spent hours listening to her songs. He brought me Virginia Woolf, Aldous Huxley and Robert Graves. He would talk a blue streak about a book and its author and leave it for me to read. I read some great books that Lennie brought over– books that made me stretch my mind as I struggled to understand. And Lennie talked all sorts of philosophical talk about politics, war and peace. And Women! He loved to talk about Women. He liked to talk about Peggy Ann and Bette Jean. Peggy hated Lennie because he was older and more worldly than she was and wise to her ways. He'd yank her covers off and make her mad. They were alike in one way; they both liked to flirt and tease. She would turn on the Charm and the boys fell under the spell of her seductive manner every time. She would catch their eye and as soon as they made a move on her she would drop them. She'd go after other girls' boyfriends and once she had them in her net, she would dump them. Boys would beg and plead for a date and she would tease them and ridicule them behind their backs and brag to the other girls how easy it was to get the boys and then brush them off.

When Peggy Ann got voted "The Prettiest Girl" in her Senior Class, Ma said, "You're playing with fire! You'll pay the Piper one day!" Peggy would pridefully toss her head ignoring Ma's words and Ma would repeatedly call her *Scarlett O'Hara*, which was understandable because Peggy Ann and cousin Bette Jean were like characters out of *Gone With the Wind*–Peggy like the saucy, egotistical and vain Scarlett and Bette Jean as the sweet, innocent Melanie. Ma and Dot Flynn were all over their daughters with criticism, multiple corrections and specious forms of encouragement. And with Peggy cast in the lead role in the Senior play and Bette Jean selected Queen of the annual *Winter Carnival Ball*, both mothers had a fertile field of unfulfilled dreams to cultivate and bring to fruition. Ma criticized Peggy to her face, but couched among her words and comments was constant verbal support for being "the vixen!" which arose naturally because she was one herself. And Dot Flynn passionately (vehemently) making up for her own mothers lack of attention to her, meticulously managed every hair on her daughters head–priming and guiding every facet of her existence to an uncomfortable place beyond exceptional. Both girls, having such honors bestowed on them with no grasp of the ultimate significance or non-significance of it all, it was only a matter of time before the two mothers were in near to open warfare about whose daughter was top doggy. As a result, the girls themselves were unwittingly set at war with each other on a permanent basis, from which neither of them ever fully recovered from the damage it did to their souls and real selves.

Bette Jean lived out Dot Flynn's fantasies and Peggy lived out Ma's fantasies. After all, we grew up on Ma's stories of herself as "The Best Dressed Girl in West Lynn." Ma told all the old boy friend stories over and over. How easy it was for her to "get the boys" and how difficult it was for her poor friend, Ann Marie.

Lennie watched it all develop and let me know with a complicit wink that he saw and understood what was going on. I liked Lennie because he would pull their covers off and say what I didn't know how to say. Peggy would walk up the stairs and catch a glimpse of Lennie's twinkling eyes, as he quipped, "You're beautiful, Baby," tossing hollow kisses across the room at her. I loved the knowing and friendly mockery in Lennie's words–loved the way the words would get to Peggy in a way that anything I might say wouldn't get to her. Peggy looked down on Lennie with utter contempt and disgust and he saw through Ma, too. He saw her for the flirt she was and saw Peggy reflected in Ma's starry eyes. Peggy and Bette fulfilled their mothers' dreams. They became their mothers' fantasies and both married men their mothers chose for them. Peggy married Paul Murphy, because Ma liked him and how religious he was, and Bette Jean, Queen of the Ball, married Peter, *King* of that same *Winter Carnival Ball* and Captain of the Football team, who Aunt Dot chose for Bette when she learned that he was going to go to Tufts University and his family was much better off financially than her own. Peggy and Bette were so competitively driven, they could not be normally happy as adults. Both had three children and later on both became divorced from their mother's pre-selected husbands.

Lennie was attracted to tall, wealthy women. His step mother, Elsie, told him, "It's as easy to love a rich girl as it is to love a poor girl." Lennie took her words to heart, found, fell in love with and married a rich girl. He met Joanne who was a senior at Regis College. She was a tall and beautiful brunette, smart and from a rich family. And to top it off, Lennie loved Joanne a lot. Ma couldn't believe how Lennie attracted such Beautiful Girls. I know why. There was something rich inside Lennie that drew ladies to him. And Elsie had bred him to be charming–a cultured gentlemen in a *Tom Jones* sort of way. Influenced possibly by F. Scott Fitzgerald, he assumed the role of the beautiful and the damned in the *Leisure Class*. Bill McKay had about as much non-use for Lennie as Dad did. And Ma said he was just using us to get away from school. He would panic when the phone rang and tell Ma not to let Elsie know he was there. "If that's Elsie..." he'd say, and put a finger over his lips and shake his head. He told tall tales–woven tales about himself. About jobs he had, people he knew and things he did. He would get fired from all of his jobs. Or he'd quit. I knew some of Lennie's stories were made up, but I liked the way he told his stories and I was a good audience for him. When Lennie was in high school, Elsie was Chairperson of the School Committee and he was a constant embarrassment to her. She was grateful when he finally got out of school. Of course, when school was no longer the issue, the job, or the lack of one, was. Elsie said that he would probably always need a woman to support him.

I learned a lot from Lennie. He created, spontaneous and fruitful leisure time with and for me and spent lots and lots of time with me. And he continued to bring me books–books I never ceased to love–*BRAVE NEW WORLD, 1984, ORLANDO*. In our many, many discussions Lennie helped validate for me much of what I was experiencing but couldn't name.

Lennie married Joanne after she got pregnant. He married her at St. Pat's because she was Catholic. Elsie was Protestant, so Lennie was Protestant, too, but mostly he was a free thinker. Ma said he did the right thing by Joanne. Ma went down to St. Pat's the Friday night Lennie and Joanne got married. She was one of a handful who witnessed their marriage. Lennie loved Joanne. He sang her praises. I liked her, too. She was quiet and pretty. They shared a deep appreciation of each other. Joanne was a teacher and got a job teaching third grade in Saugus. They had four kids and Joanne supported Lennie most of the time. They've lived in Ipswich for years and years. He worked now and then. They've been together now for thirty years. The kids are grown up. Every now and then I hear from Lennie. He came by at Christmas dressed as Santa Claus a few years before Ma died. The white beard was his own.

Nobody Ever Talked About How They Got It

Every six weeks on Thursdays, winter and summer, I went to the Polio Clinic and saw Doctor Grice. I loved him and always looked forward to seeing him. He continued to challenge me to work hard and purposely regain the greatest amount of physical function possible. He called forth the very best that was in me.

And Miss McGinnis was still (always) there in her long white coat and red painted fingernails. I never saw what it was that kept her so busy. She would stand with her arms folded in front of her and say things I would struggle to comprehend. I missed her when I didn't see her, but don't ever remember her not being there–around somewhere, with her gravel voice and sandy brown hair. Her red lipstick matched the red nail polish. She wasn't especially pretty, but did her best to emphasize what prettiness she did have with make-up. I remember watching her walk way down the long corridor. I felt lonely. Not ever really satisfied with our visits. Not really understanding the purpose of her presence. I knew what Miss Wentworth's job was, and Doctor Grice's and all the Physical Therapists, but I didn't understand Miss McGinnis's job. I had the idea that I needed someone to be there for me and somehow I attached this function to her, probably because it didn't quite fit anyone else. Each time I wanted her to stay longer than she did. When I was a full time patient, she came by every single day and never missed a day. I looked forward to seeing her and waited for her with fond expectations and hope. Her visits usually were kept to a short five minutes. We didn't have much to say to each other beyond a casual hello, because I knew that she really didn't want to hear what I wanted to say, like how hard it was for me to be there–how sad it was for me to need to be there and how lonely I felt. I wanted to tell her how hard it was for me to pretend all the time. I really wanted to tell her everything. I wanted to tell her about Timmy. How I got polio from playing naked with him in the woods. I wanted to tell her how awful I felt after I played with Timmy, because I knew we weren't supposed to look at each other's bodies and especially we weren't supposed to look at each other's bodies and touch them. That's what I never talked about. Nobody ever talked about how they got Polio. Nobody ever wanted to tell. But I knew how everybody got Polio and I knew why nobody ever told anybody. I got Polio because me and Timmy touched each other and used to pee on each other.

Timmy would put his penis between my legs and he'd pee and I'd pee and that's how I got Polio and that's what I could never tell and that's what I wanted to tell Miss McGinnis or Miss Wentworth, but if I did, I knew that they would be so surprised, shocked, so awfully disgusted that they would never again have anything more to do with me. And all the other people who had Polio would deny it. They'd say, "Oh, no. Not me!" And then it would look like it was just me and everyone would go away–Miss McGinnis and Miss Wentworth, too and I'd be all alone, ashamed, lonely and sad.

So I had to pretend I didn't know either. Miss McGinnis came in and sat beside my bed, saying serious and polite things and then she would get up and leave and I felt lonely because I still didn't have a chance to say what I really wanted to say. Other times I wanted to tell her how much I hated it when Ma and Dad came. How I hated visiting hours when they came to visit. When they would come in and sit there and we had nothing to say to each other. Miss McGinnis called them my kin-folk and I didn't like that either. I wanted to tell her I was happier in the hospital than I ever was at home. It was warmer and closer and I would be happy to stay there for the rest of my life.

I really wanted to say all of that to her, but when I tried to tell her anything real, she would say, "Oh no, you don't feel that way. You feel this way." It was no use. She just didn't get it. I couldn't find a way to connect with her as much as I hoped I would–just never did.

Years later, when I was actually enrolled at B.U. she came over there to see me every few weeks. It was such a relief for her to do that because B.U. was so horrendously huge and I was so small. When she came over I felt safe– like I could make it work.

Like before, I wanted to tell her how scared I was–how ungodly terrified– how stupid I was–how terribly shy I was and that I didn't know how to make friends or to say smart things in class. I wanted to tell her what a fraud I was and that I didn't belong there. But she heard none of it. Miss McGinnis thought it was just fine that I was there at B.U. As far as she was concerned, I was right where she unquestionably always knew I would be–getting a Liberal Arts education at Boston University, where the architect had designed those "fudgy towers." She always called them "fudgy towers"–not beautiful Gothic towers liked the ones her father had designed for Boston College. Miss McGinnis could be a snob in such matters. And at other times I felt embarrassed because I knew she felt my disease. She hurt deep down inside herself for my inside hurt. I wanted to tell her that I was aware that she had those deep down inside hurts too, because she would sometimes without knowing it, show me that she knew–really knew how hard it was for me. I saw the sadness in her eyes and in her stillness, between her formal impersonal words. That's when I'd hide and pretend not to notice. Because if I did, I'd cry for sure. And if I cried she'd pull back and make believe there was nothing to cry about, nothing to feel bad about. Somehow I had to get on with it. So there was no use in telling her all the things I wanted to tell her. So I never did. And all along, deep inside of her, she knew my sadness matched her sadness and my loneliness matched her loneliness and if either one of us ever said it out loud, we both would start to cry and never stop.

New Beginnings

In the spring of 1956 I was seventeen. Peggy was twenty and planning to marry Paul Murphy in July. Ma was thoroughly engaged, happy and excited about making the Wedding plans. A seamstress, Mrs. Blinn from Oak Street had agreed to make the Bridesmaid gowns and the Reception was to be held at Suntaug in Lynnfield. Their High school jealousies mostly behind them, Bette Jean was to be Peggy's Maid of Honor. Ma said it will be Peggy's day and if I were her Maid of Honor I would take attention away from her. So it was decided that Bette Jean would be Maid of Honor. Believe you me, I was pleased with that decision, because I didn't feel close to Peggy and I couldn't see myself side by side with her in such a grown up way. Anyhow, I had my own pre-occupation that Spring and mischievously opined to myself that what was going on with me might steal a bit of the Spotlight away from Peggy's big day.

Doctor Grice had come up with a wonderful plan to strengthen my left hand by transplanting some healthy muscles from my legs to places where the muscles didn't work, which could result in a left hand that was functional. If I was ever to fulfill my intense need to learn how to drive a car and so many other important things that could put me on the road to real freedom, I needed to be able to extend my fingers and grasp things with that hand. I had strong wrist extensors, functioning elbow flexors and my right hand was good as gold, so for months he and I planned it out. When I saw Doctor Grice at the Polio Clinic he would sit beside me, give me a wink, take my hand with sureness in his and seek out all the muscles that didn't work and showed me where he would place the new ones and how he would do that. We were such a good team. He had the vision, courage and expertise and I had the trust and willingness to make it work.

So while all the excitement of planning Peggy's Wedding was going on at home, I was hospitalized in April. The surgery was done without much ado and it was a complete success–a well deserved Olympic triumph for Doctor Grice and his team. My hand needed time to heal before physical therapy would ultimately re-train the muscles to do new jobs.

As I recovered from the surgery I was able to observe the others in my section. Across from me there was a girl who had undergone Orthopedic surgery and was barely visible under the elaborate display of traction. She looked lost in her bed under the overhead traction frame, surrounded by multiple poles, ropes, pulleys and sandbags which were overwhelming and agony for her to endure.

In the early evening the doctors who had put it all together during the day, arrived with Doctor Grice. Doctor Grice checked out the setup. His brilliance and extensive experience instantly gave him a clear vision of what was needed. He turned toward the young residents who jumped to silent attention as Dr. Grice paced around the bed and delivered firm instructions: "Take THAT down! Get rid of THAT! Remove THAT And THAT! Get rid of THAT! And THAT! And That!" Large and small pieces of the apparatus began to pile up on the floor–poles, ropes, pulleys and sandbags. And the girl in the bed began to appear again. Pretty soon there was just the traction frame with one pole going the length of the bed, a couple of ropes, a pulley and a sandbag. All so simple now. Doctor Grice looked at each and every individual doctor directly in the eye. He growled, "AND IT WORKS DAMMIT!!!".

I was thrilled and excited and a tiny bit frightened by the performance of this brilliant and demanding man. I loved him to pieces. He was my hero. I tried hard to keep up with him. To be all I could be. To match wits with him. He glowed and showed me off and took pride in my strides toward physical rehabilitation.

Many years later, in the late 1960's, I heard Hans Kung, a German Theologian, speak at the New England Life Hall in Boston. I was thrilled by that man's brilliance. He talked about stripping the Catholic Church of all that was not essential. To strip it bare of all the encumbering rules and regulations, doctrines and dogmas, until we re-discover the essence, the man, Jesus of Nazareth. I was thrilled by the simplicity of Kung's faith and his ability to express his vision in simple terms. He did to belief what Doctor Grice did in his medical work. They were both able to strip away all that was not essential.

In 1973, my Friend and grammar school teacher at St. Pats, Connie Marquis and I toured Florence, Italy. We were visiting a museum to see Michelangelo's DAVID and many of his unfinished sculptures. Connie and I were thrilled by the wonderfulness of DAVID. We stayed a very long time and listened to the tour guides talk about the great artist. There was an unfinished PIETA and MOSES (several unfinished MOSES). The tour guides explained Michelangelo's process of going out to the marble quarries in search of just the right piece of marble. He searched the quarry until he found the piece of marble that he intuitively knew contained within it the form he wanted to recreate. He brought the large piece of marble back to his workplace and began. His task was to strip this huge piece of marble of all that wasn't essential to the form–until there it stood–alive and independent–DAVID. MOSES. THE PIETA. Like Kung and Dr. Brice. I was thrilled to the deepest part of my very soul to incorporate that same process into my own development. In fact, it became my work and life ethic.

Incrementally, I gained confidence by observing how others around me did their jobs and constructed mental images of myself doing that same job or function, even better than the people I observed. I saw myself not as better than them, or more intelligent, but more of a technician learning a trade, but not necessarily inhibited by the same cultural barriers that limited them.

For so many years, I watched Miss McGinnis do her job as a Social Worker whose position was funded by the National Foundation for Infantile Paralysis. At Children's Hospital, she was part of "the team" made up of doctors, nurses and physical therapists. Miss McGinnis stood amongst them during *Grand Rounds* (teaching tool and the various rituals of medical education and inpatient care) but always a slight distance, apart, aloof, observing, commenting. Never quite connecting with me or with what I needed and wanted then. I saw me doing that job better. I knew I could do the job better because I would listen, hear, respect, love and guide the person. Make suggestions and help make dreams come true. I would not be on the side of "Grand Rounds". I would be on the side of the patient. I watched all of the women–Miss McGinnis, Miss Wentworth, Elsie MacKay, Mrs. Heath, Mrs. Elliott, Aunt Dot, Ma and Ma's friend, Molly Ahern. Ma admired Molly because she knew how to make do with very little and she set a lovely table with pretty tea cups. Women Roll Models. Ma voiced her admiration for each of those women and saw herself as not quite measuring up. They were strong and determined women. I observed each of them, Ma along with the rest. I watched Peggy Ann and Bette Jean. I watched Connie Elliott. I watched. And I thought about the kind of woman I wanted to be and what I would select from each of them to achieve that goal. I would take Miss Wentworth's gentle, compassionate love. Mrs. Heath's wisdom and appreciation of Nature, Mrs. Elliott's ability and willingness to take the time to solve problems.

And there was Molly's simplicity and Ma's willingness to do what she had to do, no matter what. But most of all, because this was my closest existential facet and although I began to view all of that at the time as a form of apprenticeship, I must admit, I did want Miss McGinnis's job.

I knew I didn't want to be like Peggy Ann or Bette Jean. There was something about being pretty and popular that hurt my stomach. I admired Mrs. Heath because she was tuned into the same things Dad noticed–the grass when it turned green in Springtime, a flowering bush, the beauty of a snow flake, a poem, an act of kindness or wisdom displayed. I admired her wisdom. I wanted to have wisdom. I wanted to have compassion. I wanted to feel and be real with, rather than simply observe, others.

I kept a notebook of famous quotations that I found in *The Saturday Evening Post, Reader's Digest* and elsewhere. I wrote letters to my friends at Children's Hospital. I wanted to go to school and Miss McGinnis talked about a Hospital School in Canton where students with disabilities lived and went to school and got medical treatment. And there was a commuter's school in Boston for students with disabilities.

But most of all, my mind was centering around the brand new high school in Stoneham where my classmates from St. Pat's were getting ready to enroll. But no one seemed to know just what to do with me. I wrote to the Superintendent of Schools and I wrote away to correspondence schools.

There was a hesitancy non-expressed and expressed by the Superintendent of the Stoneham public schools, about safety and fire laws. I would be the only student in a wheelchair, after all. Ma and Dad and I visited the Hospital School in Canton and realized it was not for me because I was able to function at home and didn't need constant medical care.

Between Doctor Grice and Miss McGinnis and the willingness of the local School Board to pay for my transportation, it was decided that I would go to the Industrial School in Boston in the Fall of 1956.

I didn't know its full title until I was driven there at nine in the morning and opened a small, very old algebra book with a book plate on the inside cover that read: PROPERTY OF THE INDUSTRIAL SCHOOL FOR CRIPPLED AND DEFORMED CHILDREN. I stared at those words for several long moments and gripping that small book tightly in my hand I looked around at that archaic city school building on St. Betolph Street with the wrought iron bars on the windows. The whole environment looked like it had been lifted out of the pages of *Oliver Twist*. I was scared to death.

Everything began at nine am. I was taken into a darkened, musty smelling room, where someone tested my eyes, hearing and speech patterns for reasons that were not explained to me. Then there was a typing class and later they had me sewing hems on dish towels that a lady said were for some charity. The building was dark and cold and all the students were severely disabled, crippled and deformed, so grotesque I felt sick–very unlike the idea I had of me. A boy, dribbling from his mouth and nose, came over to me smiling and eager to make friends. He was unable to speak and he struggled to talk. Lunch was in a basement room with long tables and small windows set high in the brick walls with wires over them. I sat staring at my lunch bag, unable to eat. I stayed still and quiet. Never before or since have I been that frightened in my entire life. When the taxi came to pick me up and bring me home it was only 2:30 and the teacher said "Good night," a strange remark to be made in the middle of the afternoon.

That night, I sat up in bed crying loudly. Ma and Dad came running in startled. I talked and cried nonstop, insisting that I would not go back there the next day, or ever. Ma paid attention. Neither of them had ever seen me that scared and upset. She agreed with me that I would not go back there. Dad said so, too. I didn't see myself as crippled or deformed. Whatever Polio meant to each of us, we, individually and as a unit were unwilling to believe or accept that the reality I experienced at The Industrial School included me. The next day Ma called Miss McGinnes and told her I would not return to The Industrial School. Miss McGinnis expressed her disappointment and said I should go back and give it a fair try.

She and Doctor Grice had supported this plan and they both insisted that I should not make up my mind so quickly. She said there were "deeper" reasons why I was resisting and we should think about those "deeper" reasons. But our deeper reasons created a united resistance and although it was a departure from the norm for all of us. It was the only time we said no to Doctor's Orders. And there were consequences to our disobedience.

Doctor Grice was extremely dissatisfied–even angry about it. He had backed that original decision for me and the expectation was that I would comply with that decision. There were issues that ran deeper than deep for me and for Ma and for Dad and also issues ran deep for Doctor Grice and Miss McGinnis. There was possibly a loss of face here, in that we should question their professional judgment– something in their minds that bordered on an insurrection. I don't know for sure. Perhaps it was simply an easy solution to a difficult problem. Through it all, I kept insisting that I could go to Stoneham High School. It was a brand new building, just two stories high. Our friend Bill Crosby was the Chief of the Stoneham Fire Department and he intervened when the Superintendent and the School Principal objected to having me at school because me and my wheelchair would be a fire hazard. Bill assured the School Board that the Fire Department would have a copy of my class schedule and would be responsible for me in case of fire.

The truth of the matter was that Stoneham High School personnel, from the School Committee members to the Superintendent, down to the Principal and Vice-Principal did not want me there. In their minds, it would have been easier for them if I went to Boston, even if the School Department paid for the taxi and the tuition, to keep me there–easier than having me attend classes in my wheelchair. Eventually, I imagine fearing public exposure of one sort or another, or a possible lawsuit, the local school officials finally agreed, to let me in, as long as I could produce a Doctor's Letter saying I was physically able to attend classes at Stoneham High.

Doctor Grice refused to write it. And he refused to see me when I visited the Clinic every six weeks. I saw other doctors who were not as involved with me as he had always been. I believed I was being punished because I would not follow his advice and go to the Industrial School. So I had to stay home all that Fall. Then finally, in February of 1957, he saw me and gave me a letter and I remember his piercing words as he stormed out of the room, "They want her to be normal and she's not normal!" The door slammed shut behind him and his flowing white coat. I felt his harsh and painful words deeply inside of me and I had to cut them off, so they would not paralyze my dreams.

So that one day at the Industrial School changed the entire course of my life and as much as it hurt, I discovered that Dr. Grice and seventeen year old me had something significant in common–a strong will and stamina. Yes, we were a pretty darn good match. And that Spring, I started at Stoneham High school as a Sophomore.

Finally a Goal!

Mr. Nadeau, the Principal and Mr. Horton, the Vice-Principal, numbly went along with my arrival. Here I was, seventeen, but felt like the ten year old I was in the 5th grade at St Pats, when I left school for summer vacation, caught the Polio and then seven years later, while I was picking up the sticks of my life as a sophomore, my old classmates from St. Pat's were Seniors.

I stayed very quiet. Very still, like the girl who was quiet and noticed all the shades of green in the grass. I studied hard and did very well on my papers and on my tests. Jane Lasalle made friends with me. Everything went slowly, very slowly, in slow motion. I went to school every day by taxi. Kids, assigned by the teachers, pushed me from class to class and gradually I made other friends. Most of my old classmates from Grammar School seemed very sophisticated and grown up–Ann Harrigan. Karen Kelly. Mary Hammel. Sally Donahue. I would watch them as I ate lunch with them in the cafeteria, but when I was with them, I still felt ten years old. At the same time there was a depth being created inside of me. A kind of maturity was happening from the inside out. Yes, back in school for the first time in seven years, I was emotionally and socially ten, but all of those years sitting in the backyard in Spring, Summer and Fall had created another mature pathway to my soul. I felt a deepness inside of me that was different from how I felt in the cafeteria or when I was being pushed along the crowded corridors. I believed in myself in a way that had been unknown and unseen by me in the prior seven years. Deep inside of me was a gradual awareness and understanding–a firmer belief in myself–a determined energy to move forward. I knew I had to do it and could do it.

It brought to mind again and refreshed again those wise words by Thoreau and Emerson: Thoreau, "Man's capacities have never been measured. No one knows what he can do. Nor are we to judge what he can do by any precedents, so little has been tried." And Emerson, "Every man is new in Nature. No one knows what he can do. Nor does he know until he has tried." Yes, socially and emotionally I was ten, but on a deeper level a Wisdom was emerging. A Wisdom that told me I was in the process of becoming. I thought then: "I am not just a Human Being! I am a Human in the process of Being!

School work didn't come easily for me, I had to work enormously hard. I loved Literature, History and Biology, but Math scared me to death. My brain froze when numbers were in front of me. In Algebra class I never balanced a single equation! Foreign Language was hard, too. My memory was of Grammar School where the Nuns were critical and punishing so I stayed very still–very quiet. I continued to observe and listen and kept on going. The guidance counselor, Mrs. Costello, didn't know what to do with me because I had no prerequisites–no classes since 5th grade and here I was seven years later in the 10th grade. I knew some of my friends were taking College courses so I took what they were taking–English, Latin, History, Math and Biology. At least I had a clear goal to aim for. I wanted to go to Boston University. It was Meaningful. It was Marvelous. It was Measurable. It was Manageable. FINALLY! A GOAL!

At first, Teachers didn't know how to deal with me. Some were overly condescending, offering far more help than I needed. Others didn't see me sitting in their classroom. The kids saw to it that I had my turn when Mr. Lamson in History class skipped over me. They just stopped and looked at me, until he noticed me. In Math class one day an announcement came over the Public Address system for all classes to report to the Auditorium.

The teacher instructed the class to proceed and then turned to me and said I should wait there in the classroom. Shortly, two Firemen came into the room, carefully examining the closets and drawers. "A bomb scare," they said. Not to worry. They were quite sure it was a false alarm. I was stunned to think I had been left behind to blow up.

Mary Larange became my friend. She worked at the *Arnold House* nursing Home on William Street with Ma and Aunt Dot. She took the risk one day and said "Hello." She brought me into her group of friends, and they gave me support and encouragement by accepting me as one of them. These friends, Robin, Brenda, Toby, Marsha, Mary Jo, Carol, Wilma, and Ione, each showed me the way and I followed them willingly and gratefully.

By the time I graduated in June of 1959 the school personnel was very much at ease with me, mainly because I was smart and did my work really well. The 10th Graders did a "This Is Your Life" show for me in the Spring of 1959. The Auditorium was filled with my peers. I sat on stage with Ma and Paul and Elsie MacKay and Earle Potter (my taxi driver) and the 10th Graders read letters from Doctor Grice and even Peggy, who was taking care of her new baby. I was graduating from Stoneham High School and for two hours, one afternoon, time stood still and noticed me. When I graduated from Stoneham High School I was a star. A celebrity. "That was MY LIFE! I got lots of awards and honors and scholarships to go to Boston University. Even Mr. Nadeau and Mr. Horton congratulated me. They shook my hand and said they would miss me.

Meanwhile, at home, I still found myself coming from the place of being a sick child–a victim of Polio. Only a quasi-physical Survivor. I still felt shame and humiliation in my child-body–a body that did not mature on the surface–a body that did not take the shape and form of adulthood. I ate very little and stayed very thin. There continued to be no way to take in more nourishment at home. I saw my classmates and neighborhood friends, Ann Harrigan, Karen Kelly, Tommy Elliott and Jackie grow up, while I stayed the same. As they grew up I saw less and less of them. I stayed behind, trapped in my child-body. Ma continued to take care of me. Earl Potter was the taxi driver who took me to school every day. He lifted me in and out of the car as I still was not yet able to transfer independently. Earl didn't talk much, but I knew he was a good friend. On Memorial Day he came and got me and took me to the Parade. I stayed in the car and watched the Parade and thought Earl was a good man and so patient. His sons were classmates of both me and Peggy.

On Sunday mornings I had a complete bed bath. Ma brought a basin of warm water and placed it on a towel by my side so I could wash myself. Then she would come in and wash my back and my feet. We had built a partial bath in my new room with a toilet and sink but without a shower or tub. In the 1950's the idea of independent living for people with disabilities hadn't yet emerged and Ma and Dad still thought of me as their ten year old sick child. Mary Larange and Wilma Graham often came to see me on Sunday mornings after Mass. Usually they arrived before I had a chance to get dressed and I visited with them in my pajamas. I liked their visits and we had good conversations, but the feeling of being a sick child visited by friends bothered me, especially since in so many other ways, we were equals. Ma had her way of being grateful to them for coming by that left a residue of shame inside of me because she was unable to accept the fact that I actually had friends–not just dutiful acquaintances who only came by because they felt sorry for the sick child. I carried that sick child feeling inside of me through high school and college. My life centered around attending classes and coming home to study and be taken care of. Part of me was terrified that I was a fraud–that I had no business in the classroom–that I belonged at home... forever the sick child locked into a mentality of suffering, accepting one's cross. After all, God listens to the prayers of a sick child. Ma talked about "dragging that wheelchair around" when we had opportunities to go out. She knew other people did not want to drag that wheelchair around and politely declined many invitations for me to go out and be with kids from school. Some became persistent. Some were able to break though Ma's resistance. I wanted to be with Robin and Toby and Brenda. I went to the Movies with Brenda and her mother, Mrs. Boyle, to see "South Pacific" at the Granarda Theater in Malden. It was the first time since I had Polio that I went to the Movies and I was both excited and intimidated by the crowd of people in the Theater. I remember looking around and feeling awed just being there. Brenda lifted me in and out of the car, folded my wheelchair and put it in the trunk. Marsha was tiny, but she was able to lift me into the car, too, when we went shopping together. My own expectations and the expectations of my family were so different from the norm, but I have come to bless that difference. But I still felt diminished– a paralyzed infant with no sexuality–no expectation that I would have boy friends, or date, or marry and have children. It seemed like I would be an un-walking age ten forever.

Today, in my work as a Mass Rehabilitation Counselor, I see families struggling with those same issues of "independent functioning" for their adult disabled children. I see the same "caring for" in so many families and I encourage them to know that their lives can be different. The disability issues are among many in the family system of issues, personalities and needs.

But even with those lingering and intense feelings of discontent and resistance, I took some solace in being aware that I was still on the path of finding my way out. I sought and found the quietness deep down inside–that familiar place of refuge and safety and the realness of me being alive beneath the radar of the child-body. I remember sitting in that space of my room on a Sunday afternoon–going deep down inside into the stillness, seeking and experiencing the essential quietness of that space. Dad and Ma were in the living room after Sunday dinner. I was teaching at St. Pats at that time and would go to my room to prepare the lesson plans for the week ahead. I would take my book with pictures and words and memories–hold the book open and sink deep, deep down into that timeless area–and after a long time in that space I'd come alive for all the work I needed to do. I remember becoming aware that if God wanted me to be doing anything else, He would show me how. A person or opportunity would emerge. All I needed to do was keep my mind open and alert to see the sign when it appeared. Like the wise virgins who kept the lamps burning so they'd know when their time came. There were lots and lots of Sunday afternoons spent that way–alone, deep down inside of myself, with Life.

In April 1958, when I was eighteen, I had the final surgery–the last piece of physical rehabilitation left to do. It was the last of my work with Doctor Grice. He had accepted a position at the University of Pennsylvania Medical

School as Chief of Orthopedic Surgery to begin July 1st. Our work together was complete. Together we had brought my physical rehabilitation to its maximum potential. I had walked across the room and back. And this surgery for the final functional restoration of my left hand. Two years earlier I had the muscle, which meant now I had a more normal floppy wrist. That was the deal, finger flexors for a floppy wrist and now to stabilize the wrist required a bone graft which took bone from my pelvis to my wrist. My left thumb had flexibility, but not extension so the surgery included a graft to give me a stable, oppositional thumb. After years of mindful planning and the two surgeries, finally I would have a fully functional left hand–a stabilized wrist and fingers that could open and close, including a thumb that could complete a grasp. I was hospitalized again in the six bed ward on Division 25. I awakened after surgery with pain in the palm of my hand that was unequal to any physical pain I ever had before, or since. For two days, pain medication was withheld because my breathing was too shallow to tolerate the medication. I remember the pain and tears and the deep sense of self-awareness. The pain in my hand was sharp and deep and unrelenting, burrowing a hole through the palm from one side to the other. My left hand is very special to me.

I hold it as a sacred work of belief in human potential. It is a work of art, created (recreated) by Doctor Grice and me. Together we constructed a functional hand along with deep pain and deep joy, simultaneously. Today I hold my left hand with grateful appreciation in the palm of my right hand, always the stronger of the two, and I cherish all of the memories of all of the days, of all of the years of care, hope, excitement and pain finally resulting in the re-creation of its essential usefulness. Today that hand controls the acceleration and the breaking in my van–all the horsepower that takes me to all the places of work and play. And it's that hand that rests my head as I lean onto that side at night and during the day.

I rest my chin on the curved fingers of my precious left hand. And over and over and over I give thanks to God and Doctor Grice and myself for all the brilliance and willingness and bravery it has taken to be here now.

***

I knew it. Deep in my gut, I knew it. I didn't know it, but I KNEW. I SURELY KNEW.

It was Tuesday, October 4th 1960. I was a sophomore at B.U. taking Political Science. On the 6:30 WBZ-TV News, it was announced that Eastern Airlines Jet Flight 375, EnRoute to Philadelphia, had crashed in Boston

156

Harbor on takeoff from Logan Airport. 62 passengers were missing and presumed dead.

I knew but said nothing. I went to school the next day. But I knew. I just knew. And when I came home Ma said, "... the plane crash..." I knew. I just knew. "Sally Arnold called"... did I know? ... Yes, I knew... I mourned for him... more deeply than I ever could have known. I grieved the loss of a great man and my dear friend... Dr. Grice.

PART THREE

B.U. (Be You)

In 1959 the only college in the Boston area that offered wheelchair accessibility was Boston University. None of the State colleges at Boston, Salem or Lowell were wheelchair accessible. BU also had a Home-to-School telephone tutorial program for students unable to attend classes. It was that program Miss McGinnis knew about. She knew its Director, Mrs. Gambel, her BU contact whom she had told me about years before. She introduced me to Mrs. Gambel, who realized immediately that I was capable of actually attending classes. Miss McGinnes had planted the seed. "BU," she said. "Some day, BU." The seed had taken root. I flourished.

I continued to be very quiet–watching and noticing.

"Yes, it is a lovely reality when someone's dream is loved into being" especially when it is mine.

Miss McGinnis had showed me the way out. Ahead of me she glanced back over her shoulder and said, "This way. Come this way." She walked on ahead and I followed. Today, February 13, 1995, we postponed our luncheon visit to the Museum of Fine Arts for the third time because of the perils of Winter. But we're on now for next month. Funny how we re-found each other again, after so many years in between. The year I turned fifty I looked her up along with other people significant to the happy place I found myself in 1989. We had left off in 1969 when she wanted to write a book using letters I'd written to her to show the process of recovery following Polio and to support her thesis that individuals who develop a disability in childhood also develop compensatory potential for success later in life. I didn't want to collaborate then–afraid my voice was not quite ready to be heard and her voice reflected her perception of events that did not reflect mine. I discovered her twenty years later writing her own story, as I had embarked upon writing mine. Two strong women now able to sit side by side and share our journeys. Two souls now meeting on a common pathway and not finished yet. There was and still is something left for us to learn from each other. We were born into different life circumstances–lived very different lives. My blue collar upbringing contrasted sharply with her family of influence privilege and opportunity. Yet there are things that have brought us together in sameness. She left her career in Music to be a Social Worker for the National Foundation for Infantile

Paralysis in the late 1940's and early 1950's at Children's Hospital. She had both intention and training then for work and service. She carried herself deliberately, self assured and difficult not to admire. She took each day in stride with her starched stiff, long white coat which was her hospital uniform–the sleeves rolled up, revealing her tanned and braceleted arms.

Stoneham High School and my friends there had provided a weaning away of my earlier attachment to Children's Hospital, but I continued to keep my connection with Miss McGinnis through the letter writing. It was easy for me to communicate in letters–to say what I wanted to say, to think my thoughts out loud–to put myself out there without fear of self-annihilation. And I needed a strong ally as I moved beyond my family and into a life of my own, and Elizabeth McGinnis was that ally.

I struggled then to be grown up, feeling that I lagged behind. I didn't measure up to the outgoing, energetic Freshmen I encountered at Boston University. There were no "Independent Living" skill trainers then. No centers staffed with other individuals with disabilities ready to lead the way, ready to say, "This is how you do it, kid." Along with my own fears, I regularly had Ma and Dad's fears to push against. The thought of going to College had not occurred to them. They kept their sanity and their faith by their docile, dogged, day by day devotion to Duty. They kept their focus straight in front and provided a home, three meals a day, clothing and shelter and gave with all their hearts all that they had to give. But it was up to us in our situations to create our own vision, find our own star and follow where it would lead us. Miss McGinnis provided a light that led my way out. She was so unlike me in so many ways, yet it was her job that I wanted. She represented life beyond the limitations of my home and my small minded home town thinking. She was there for me in a way that was not oppressive, judgmental, or demanding. I have to admit that she brought out a competitive streak in me that I wasn't aware that I had. I had to reach out and ask for her to be there and when I did she was. There was wisdom and strength in that relationship, more than I realized then, and some frustration in our clash of backgrounds as well. I didn't want to be dependent on her. Luckily I was never in love with her. Not that emotions shamed me, or pushed me away. I liked her and found her ways interesting. Her language was different–so many words I didn't know. Words that sounded sophisticated, distant, cool, detached. But she had been there from the beginning–standing with her arms folded in front of her, back on her heels in her heavy oxfords. "Bum feet" she said, which kind of put her in league with the rest of us, I guess. Not much else of her life experience did. She was rightfully proud of her father's work around Boston and later in Washington, DC, where he designed the National Shrine of the Immaculate Conception.

When I graduated from Stoneham High School in June of '59, I had become a member of the National Honor Society and that following September I started at Boston University. Months of planning and especially worry over transportation was resolved when it was decided that I could live on campus. I had never lived away from home. In fact at that point in my life I had not been away from home for even a week-end, except for my stays at Children's Hospital. At BU I was assigned a single room in The Towers–the newest Women's Dorm. In retrospect, I can't imagine how I thought I could do it all by myself. To manage at The Towers, I had to be able to transfer in and out of bed and to raise myself up without difficulty. I was able to push my chair without too much difficulty, though not outdoors, but at least enough indoors to make me think I could handle it.

Ma and Dad were nervous wrecks. I was too. When we arrived at BU on that first Sunday afternoon, Dad lost his footing lifting me out of the car and we tumbled in a heap to the pavement and my ankle got sprained.

So I started my first day, like all the other Freshmen, scared, accompanied by apprehensive parents and the added caveat of a swelled up right foot. My single room was at the end of a corridor filled with excited Freshman girls (a long way from being independent women). Several of the girls came from New York and were trying hard to act sophisticated. I didn't know anyone. But I felt excited and wanted to make a go of this venture.

Ma and Dad left as soon as they had my things arranged in my room. There was lots of activity as I swam in the sea of confusion, excitement and anticipation. A sophomore boy was my mentor and took me around to do all the necessary Registration stuff. My foot swelled more and more. The next day Ma came in and soaked the foot in a basin and wrapped it with an ace bandage.

Meantime, I had awoken early to give myself all the time I needed to wash up, dress and get ready for the day. It was a bitterly cold September and Bay State Road had a wind that cut across my face. I stung on the outside and I stung on the inside. Although I moved through each day one step at a time, each step was a tremendous effort requiring all the bravery I could muster. I was alone in the world with a desperately strong intention to make life work for me.

Alone meant hailing someone to give me a push down the street to the Academic buildings, seeking out assistance in the Cafeteria, requesting that doors be held open. I was in the bathroom of the dorm one morning toward the end of my first week and I came out of the stall, rolled over to the sink, leaned back and careened out of my chair, crashing backward, slamming the back of my head on the tile floor. I had forgotten to zip-up the leather back of the chair when I transferred from the toilet to the wheelchair. I screamed as I fell and girls rushed over and helped me back into the chair and zippered the back. They helped me put ice on the gaping wound on the back of my head.

I couldn't do it. It was just too much. I wasn't equal to the enormous task of living independently. I had indeed bitten off more than I could chew. The giant step from dependency at home to independency at BU was impossible. I talked with the woman who was the Dorm mother. I talked with my Academic Advisor. I talked with Ma. And I talked with Miss McGinnis. Classes were starting and I knew if I was going to compete adequately I couldn't miss any. I went home before the first week was over. I couldn't live at BU but I knew the next step. I had to find a way to get in and out to school from home. I got lucky right away. The Guidance Staff at BU got to work on it and fixed me up with commuting students from Stoneham–Sheila Kliner and Linda, a pretty blond girl from Butler Ave, and Sam, an athletic girl, who drove, so that first semester they picked me up in the morning and drove me home in the afternoons. At that time I was unable to transfer independently from the car to my wheelchair and I had to be lifted. Sam was the strong one who lifted me in and out of the car. Since I continued to be anorexic, weighing no more than seventy-five pounds, so the chore was relatively easy for her. However other obstacles toward gaining independence afflicted me. Power equipment wasn't even a thought then. And there wasn't room in the driveway at home for my manual chair to fit beside the car and the side of the road was too uneven for transferring. Because of that, I hadn't learned to use a sliding board to transfer from the car to the chair and vice-versa, as I did from my bed. I finally learned how to do that when Ann Marois, another wheelchair student, showed me how when I spent a weekend at her home in Weston Mass. Ann came from Ohio with her brother, Luke and her Mother when her Dad took a job as a Lawyer in a Boston firm. She had Polio and was finding her way as a young woman with a disability. Ann was a student in Business Administration but more than anything she wanted to get married. Eventually, she transferred to the University of Illinois, well known at the time for wheelchair accessibility and independence for students with disabilities. She met a fellow there and married him. We stay in touch every Christmas.

For me, at that time, being at BU was stretching me to my outer limits. The thought of me going to Illinois was beyond imagining. Instead, I pushed forward, taking on the immense challenge of being where no one in my family had ever been before. Carefully scheduling classes for three days each week, I took twelve credits, four courses in the College of Liberal Arts, on Mondays, Wednesdays and Fridays. I took English Composition, English Literature, Introduction to Sociology and a course labeled "What Is Math?" I told myself to stick with the same attitude I had when I first began at Stoneham High and remembered not to worry about keeping up. I just had to continue to survive on a daily basis and do what I had to do. I found that to be a good working attitude and I made the Achievement List that semester. Three B's and a C.

Miss McGinnis had talked BU into my ear as long as I could remember. "There's nothing like a Liberal Arts Education," she said. "When the time comes I'll introduce you to Alice Gambel." It was the place I had to be. BU became "Be You." Even while I was struggling to adjust to High School, Miss McGinnis had regularly prodded me about BU. I found her vision of BU irritating because it seemed so far ahead of me–too far in the future to present a tangible reality. Although Boston University was the only Boston area college accessible to wheelchair students in the late 1950s, I went there to get a basic Liberal Arts education. Every two weeks, Miss McGinnis came over to BU from Children's Hospital. We met near the elevator and found an empty room to sit and visit. She still was my good friend and my mentor. I needed her and she was there continuing to say things that interested me–strange things I had to reach for–ideas I had to reach for. We talked about my courses–the subjects themselves– Literature, Music and Fine Arts. She knew so much more than I did–adding to and enhancing what I was learning. At that time we still hadn't got to talking about the deeper, more personal emotional stuff–all the kid stuff that was still under the surface, though some of that did come out in my letters to her–letters written between visits at BU. I don't think Miss McGinnis felt equal to that task and from time to time when I ventured forth with more painful stuff and questions about sexuality and relationships, she was quick to suggest that perhaps I should speak with a psychiatrist. That shut me up good.

Friendships

I didn't try to keep up or fit in socially at BU. I could not consider being active in that way, because it would complicate what I needed to accomplish academically and my future was too important to compromise. I loved my courses and the discussions that went on around me. All of me (or what I conceived to be all of me at that time) was being stretched to the limit. I continued to stay quiet and only rarely ventured to speak. I listened, watched and took it all in. The classes were huge. I watched as others raised their hands, asked questions and responded to questions. I never participated. I didn't want anyone to notice me and tell me I really didn't belong there. I felt like a fraud in a world I really didn't belong to. In a way, BU was like being in my family. I didn't belong there either and if I let myself be too noticed, even during my BU days, Peggy was quick to tell me to shut up–quick to tell me I didn't belong. There was this unrelenting meshing of exclusion at home and school and I struggled to push what was necessary out of me to survive in both environments and thus hold reign above it. During that extraordinary four year adventure at BU, I pushed forward from deep inside my protective barbed wire existence with my manufactured glossy smile that I felt radiated over-gladness, so I took Public Speaking and got an A. I learned that I was good at speaking when I had time ahead to plan what I wanted to say. I was terrified of speaking spontaneously and froze when I was pointed to and asked for a response. I simply said, "I don't know" and later, in my mind, recalled all the details of what I really did know, in fact. I wanted to take "Oral Inter pretation" in the Theater Arts Department, but never did simply because I wasn't able to fit it into my tight schedule. I had the idea that with the properly selected material, I was good at speaking clearly and well and that was good enough.

For all four years, my courses were scheduled for Monday, Wednesday and Friday, which meant I studied at home on Tuesday and Thursday. BU was huge–filled with people from all over the world. I loved its diversity. Crowds of students filled the elevators between classes. There was no special treatment for students with Special Needs. It was every man or woman for him or herself. At the end of class I hurried along the corridor, pushing my manual chair to the nearest elevator and waited with the others. And when the door opened I pushed forward as aggressively as the rest. I learned not to look up into their faces. I kept my head level and with a cold determination I pushed straight on board. One time I remember the elevator filled up too fast for me. I was left out of the packed car and one person said, "This isn't fair." But no one moved. The doors closed and I simply waited for the elevator to come back again.

BU was so big and impersonal, College was mostly work and no play. I would get steely eyed like a "fighter pilot" as I pushed myself from class to class. Fire doors swung open and shut at intervals along the long corridors. They swung shut behind hurrying students as I approached from behind and yelled, "Hold the door!" Sometimes they heard, slowed down and held the door. Otherwise, I waited and pushed through with the next person going my way. Occasionally as I pushed down the hallway someone would say, "Ya wanna push?" My response? Brief, but explicit, "Yeah. Great. Thanks," I ate lunch in the Lounge where I met Connie Yahimski, Joan Hollander and Judy Nichols. They became my first BU friends. They each came to my house several times although I have lost touch with them over the years. But overall it was hard for me to make more solid friendships there until I met Sharon Beavers, Ann Marois and George Brady–all wheelchair students disabled by polio and we became solid friends.

Sharon was severely disabled by Polio early in childhood. Her Dad was in the Military and her family lived all over the world. Sharon's care wasn't consistent so she didn't have the advantage of a medical team following her closely. She had a severe curvature of the spine. Although her body was small Sharon wasn't small in any other way. She had a beautiful singing voice and sang to entertain others. She had curly dark hair, expressive hazel eyes, and a quick, easy smile. I liked her friendly style very much. Sharon got married to Bill Beaber, an Air Force Captain. He was good looking and loved Sharon. Ma couldn't imagine anyone loving someone who used a wheelchair and she said Bill was only marrying Sharon for political favor with the Military. "After all, how could he love her?" she would say. I knew how. Sharon was lovely. She died a few years after their marriage from complications of a pregnancy. I missed her for a long time.

Ann Marois was also in a wheelchair because of Polio. She came to Boston with her family from Ohio. Her Dad was a lawyer and they lived in a beautiful, sprawling house in Weston, Massachusetts. Ann was tall and attractive with close cropped brown hair and large brown eyes. She was friendly and outgoing and wanted to get married more than anything. I was amazed by her self confidence and her unrelenting expectation to date and marry. I enjoyed the stretch her friendship was for me, because I felt so far out of her league–not nearly as self-confident–not nearly so sure of myself. Eventually, Ann left BU to go to the University of Illi-nois which was known for its wheelchair accessibility. I admired Ann's courage but her goals terrified me. There was nothing in my experience to support wanting to get married or moving so far away–not even in my dreams. Ann met Ciro in Illinois; they were married on Cape Cod and are still married. We write every Christmas. Ann has worked part time as an accountant and has been busy socially in her community. Like me, she now uses an electric wheelchair and has recently learned to drive a van.

My friend George. Dear George. When he died in 1969 the words that rose up in me were "Free at last! Free at last! Thank God Almighty, he's free at last!" I was thinking of how confined George was physically. He contracted Polio in 1956 when he was a junior at Malden Catholic High School. George was brilliant. He had red curly hair clear blue eyes and a light complexion. He was tall and skinny and Polio did a weird thing to him. It paralyzed him from the waist up. His legs were strong, so if someone supported his body he could stand and walk. He could stand to transfer into the car or bed. But he had a terrible time breathing and had to gulp for each breath. He would gulp in a bunch of air and seemed to swallow it. He would toss his head back as he gulped for the air. He couldn't use his hands at all–not to eat, or brush his teeth, or hold his cigarette. We became very good friends–mostly telephone friends. He'd call and each time we would talk for an hour at least. There were so many things that George loved to talk about. Politics, world history, music, opera, and art. Occasionally, we went to the Museum of Fine Arts and the Science Museum. George was the eldest of six and he loved his brothers and sisters. He kept me up to date on their active, eventful lives. And George had an incredible mother. She went to BU with him, took all his notes and helped him study. He majored in Russian and minored in Political Science. His mother took Russian herself so she could help him. After BU, George got a Master's in Russian Studies from Emmanuel. Later he did translations for several companies. When The Boston Symphony Orchestra celebrated its Golden Trumpet Ball George wrote to the Moscow Philharmonic Orchestra inviting them to participate. He translated their reply which was in the Program for the Ball. That was a highlight for George. He often attended opening night at the Symphony and opening night for the Opera, wearing a tux and all. George married Beverly, his nurse. One evening, after they had come home from a movie, George was at his typewriter with his stick in his mouth when Beverly became aware of his stillness. He had simply stopped breathing. We all mourned his loss for a long time. George was such a bright and shining star. He is alive and present in me right now as I write these words. He encourages me to write. He says, "Do it!" These friends from BU were nourishment for me as I continued to grow toward the light.

During those years at BU, my body had atrophied considerably. I was literally skin and bones–not much flesh anywhere. I wore a heavy corset to support my diaphragm and lax stomach muscles. My breasts were small, as was the rest of me with all the atrophied muscles–unable to give me shape and identity as a woman. I continued to think of myself as a girl and stayed mostly quiet, participating simply by being there, watching and listening and having thoughts of my own.

"There is nothing like a Liberal Arts education," Miss McGinnis would say so often. She was so right. I loved many of the exciting teachers I had then–Marx Wotofsky, Murray Levin, Sterling Lanier and K.M. Badger. And so I loved Philosophy, Political Science and American Literature–Walt Whitman, Shakespeare and Modern Art. I loved it all and still do up to this very day.

My Liberal Arts education at Boston University has enriched my life to my very bones. It has been the foundation for my work as a Teacher and Counselor. It stimulated my already awakened senses to the intellectual world around me. Lennie had been my first introduction to the world of higher education. And today new people and places are drawing me even further along the path of knowledge and new ideas–beckoning me forward and deepening my awareness of what it means to be fully awake and human.

Father T

Away from BU–at home, Father T's Tuesday morning visits was all I had for company. For two years, he became my friend and my one and only social life–the closest thing I had to a boy friend. Living in my child body and still being taken care of by my Ma and Dad, I couldn't imagine being capable of a romantic relationship. I was nothing like Ma or Peggy or Bette Jean. Deep down inside I felt shame as I compared myself to Ann, and Sharon and George.

They seemed so much more grown up than I was.

Father Smith had sent Father T into my orbit from Saint Patrick's Church to counter the Non-Catholic philosophical trend at BU. Father Smith had been faithful for years to his monthly visit to bring me Holy Communion and would regularly ask if I wanted to "tell the father anything," which was his way of asking if I wanted to go to Confession. I didn't. Father Smith had the idea that because Father T was very young and "close to the books" he would keep me in the fold. Our Parish at St. Pat's was Father T's first assignment following his ordination at twenty-six. He was small in stature with a slight build and penetrating brown eyes. He was already balding and his crew cut made him look boyish at the same time. His family owned a successful furniture business and he did enjoy the privilege of money and opportunity. He and his two siblings entered Religious Life. His brother, Dick, left the Seminary before ordination and chose to marry. His younger sister, Patty, was a fully professed nun and died of cancer at thirty-one. Father T liked "nice things" which included his brand new black Plymouth Fury. He enjoyed skiing in Vermont with his priest friends and talked of an A-Shaped Chalet. He and another priest friend bought a cottage on Cape Cod and had a small boat they enjoyed in summer. Our lives were very different. My pathway had taken me inward, his had taken him outward.

I looked forward to each Tuesday morning. It was a time for me away from the books and attention was focused on me. On some level there was an intimacy between us, although we rarely agreed on any specific idea or life experience. He was young, wealthy and unaware of many (if any) inward experiences, but oh how he loved that new shiny black Plymouth Fury with the white wall tires and red interior. Sometimes I couldn't believe that guy–

168

that priest–how easily he could rationalize the good life. He figured, after all, priests gave up so much else for God! So why not? A few creature comforts weren't so much to have in return. But I really couldn't believe that guy. Yet he was gentle and compassionate and listened to me intently, even though he never understood a thing I said. I came to love Father T as much as I disliked him. He was all I had at the time. But I continued to spend much of my time at home alone. Ma worked at the Arnold House three days a week with Aunt Dot. Father T's visits were consistent and dependable and I looked forward to seeing him and continuing our ongoing conversations. We were so different. I would tease him and sometimes he would get angry. I took delight in knowing I knew more about Life than he did. We met every week on Tuesday at eleven o'clock for two and a half years. "Sixteen Steps to the Church" was the thin text he brought with him which was the basis of our conversations. Months later, we were still trying to resolve the First Step! The depth of my spiritual awareness had no corresponding place in his religious experience. Although our differences were irreconcilable, he was a compassionate soul and terribly sincere in his heart. But the best thing of all, he showed up every Tuesday with all his boyish zeal.

For Ma and Dad, attending Mass on Sunday was an Obligation that did not apply to me because I was, after all, a sick child. Father T didn't see it that way and from his point of view, participating in the Mass and receiving Holy Communion among a Faithfull Community was an opportunity that should be available to me. The Church in Stoneham was not wheelchair accessible. There were many stairs leading to the Upper Church and fewer, but still many, leading to the Lower Church. Father T assured Ma and Dad that the Church Ushers would be glad to help carry me over the stairs. Taking me to Church disrupted our Sunday routine because Ma and Dad were the first to arrive on Sunday for the 7:00 o'clock Mass. Taking me, meant going later, to the 9:00 o'clock. Once inside the Lower Church, we had to find an out of the way place for me to sit, so we sat near the Confessional. Going up to the Altar Rail for Communion was not possible because the aisle was too narrow for me and others. If I wanted to receive Communion I needed to sit by myself near the Altar Rail by the Organ. Sometimes the Priest distributing Communion was aware of me and I was given Communion, but other times he was not and I was passed by. Once the new routine was established and we got serious about me going to Mass, we started to go to Saint Athanasius Church in Reading, which was new and easily accessible. Eventually, the Eucharist became an important source of Spiritual nourishment for me and Mass was never an obligation, but rather a firm and permanent communion with an adult faith community that validated my identity as a spiritual being from that time on and throughout my lifetime.

Years later, when I was teaching at St. Patrick's Grammar School, I found myself missing Father T a lot. He had left St. Pat's and Stone-ham to study *Advanced Theology* in Canada–then off to Washington, DC, with the expectation of studying in Rome, which never happened. The turbulent Sixties took him by surprise and threw him off balance. He never recovered. His tightly woven world fell apart and he became an alcoholic. After years of unsuccessful detox, he did finally get sober. I saw him when I celebrated my fiftieth birthday. Having abdicated what was left of his better self, he was hollowed out, empty and cynically disparaging of himself. But he did remain in the Priesthood and continued to teach Ethics in a Catholic Nursing School. I loved him still in an empathic, compassionate way. My life had become richly deeper and full of grateful appreciation of all that had been, all that was and all that was yet to be. Our differences reflected the paradox of what truly is and what is not opportunity in this life.

And as unlikely as it was to me at the time, Father T turned out to be the guide leading this needy soul to that deeply refreshing and renovating spiritual watering hole.

Leaving Cottage Street

It was 1963 and selling the house on Cottage Street was especially hard on Dad. The house was his pride and joy–the only home for him and his family since 1935.

And in 1963 I was twenty-two, about to graduate from college and I wondered how I was going to get on with my life at that point, because no matter how we looked at the house, it meant no easy access for me using a motorized wheelchair, which soon would be introduced into my life. And the family culture of that period unilaterally supported the idea that unmarried adult children should remain at home, thereby allowing the family unit to continue ad infinitum.

But I had other ideas. I had to get on with my life. I needed to get a job and I needed to learn to drive. Ma was willing to talk about looking for another house that would provide easier access. Dad went passive. He wanted things to remain the same. He wanted me to stay home. To just be there. He would take care of me and I'd be safe. He would take me out for a ride on Saturday afternoons. As far as Dad was concerned, I was still his little girl and he'd take care of me forever. Ma wasn't passive. She called Von O'Brien who was a Real Estate person in town. Von and Bob had lost their sixteen year old daughter to cancer the year before. Von was empathetic and knew the kind of house we needed–an accessible, three bedroom ranch. Von found lots of houses for Ma and Dad to look at, but one after the other, Dad turned them down. He continued to resist Von's advice. She was so optimistic and could always see the possibilities Dad didn't want to see. Paul was a Sophomore at Malden Catholic High that year. He didn't say anything, but I knew it was hard on him, too. He had grown up on Cottage Street. It had memories, friendships and the old apple tree.

In February 1963 the property at 150 North Street went on the market– one mile away at the other end of Oak Street, just a half mile from 25 Oak, where the Flynn's lived. It was a three bedroom ranch, with an attached garage and breezeway. There was a fireplace in the living room, a full cellar and a large, accessible back yard. The house had a sunshiny openness–airy and spacious. It had been built for a woman who used a wheelchair. She had passed away the previous November and now her husband was selling the house and moving to Florida. The house was painted PINK! Dad hated that pink! But, the house had everything else we were looking for. The hallway was extra wide. The bathroom was roomy. This was IT! But we had to sell 37 Cottage to buy 150 North Street. Dad's heart was broken. All along he really didn't think we'd find the right house. And here it was, only a short distance away from his Sister, Dot Flynn's house. But he was depressed and just sat in his chair in the living room behind the Evening Globe, not even smoking his pipe. He didn't actively oppose the move any more. He simply went passive and did nothing to help in any way. He disappeared and let Ma do all the work with Von O'Brien. We sold our house for $16,000.00 and bought the new one for $18,000.00. We moved in on June 4, 1963, the day after I graduated from Boston, University.

Ma and Dad had lived twenty-eight years at 37 Cottage Street, and it was awfully painful for Dad to leave what was his pride and his deepest sense of himself. He left the house quietly, with no words. Ma had the courage to do what needed to be done. As time went on and 150 North Street became home, Dad gradually began to love the new house. He planted a garden. He had a new work bench downstairs, room for his photo dark room and racks for his hunting guns and fishing rods. He took and developed new pictures. He painted the house blue. And for the old fishermen, Dad, Phil and Flo, getting their boat in and out of the garage was easier. Over time, he grew proud of his new home. Ma missed her neighbors and her dining room and Paul missed Cottage Street too, but I loved everything about the new house, especially the new found freedom of getting in and out all by myself and eventually I got a job, learned to transfer in and out of the car and learned to drive.

Trial & Error

In the fall of 1958, when I was a Senior at Stoneham High, I had been introduced to Paul Curry–my first Mass. Rehabilitation Counselor. Essentially, by playing the Devil's Advocate, Paul taught me Self-reliance– how to push back against resistance–how to find my way in the adult world by trial and error and above all else, how to rely on my own judgment. Mass. Rehab was then and is now the Massachusetts Public Vocational Re-habilitation Program, federally funded and mandated to assist people with disabilities toward the goal of employment. Counselors are trained to understand the various challenges encountered by disabled folk and to assist those who have potential for productive employment. The money is there for assistive technology, restoration services, training and job placement. The counselor/client relationship can be a powerful tool in the life of a person with a disability.

I have spent much time reflecting on the nature and motivation of people who chose to be counselors to people with disabilities. My impression, years ago, was that they offered resistance–presented the "what ifs" resistance that parents, teachers, friends and do-gooders had already voiced. It seemed to be my job to counter their resistance with my arguments for how I should proceed with my own life. I began to learn early on that Mr. Curry, in his role of Devil's Advocate, worked for his Agency, not necessarily for me. I was very clear about my vocational objectives. I wanted to be a Medical Social Worker (wanted Miss McGinnis's job). Mr. Curry was very clear. The goal of Mass Rehab was limited to providing undergraduate financial assistance leading to entry level employment and that goal required a Master's Degree. He discouraged my goal, offering unlimited reasons why this was not a reasonable vocational objective for me, including the reminder that Social Work schools were not accessible and internships required mobility and flexibility. If he offered reasonable alternatives, I don't remember them. I knew what I wanted and was clear in my intentions and determined to hold on to my objectives, no matter what. How that would play out, I didn't know, but I did feel that I had Mr. Curry pretty well psyched out. I needed to play his game–appear to listen to him–deliver to his ears what he wanted to hear and see, but not lose sight of my own goals, dreams and ideals, which meant back to my old defense mechanisms that had served me so well in my earlier polio days–stay quiet and don't let him see too much of me–stay invisible and inaudible. Just tell him what he needs to hear, so that I get what I need from his Agency. I had to be vigilant, because I felt that if I truly revealed myself, he would likely walk away, unwilling to assist me. So, in the face of Mr. Curry's continuing objections to my goal of Medical Social Work, I smiled my sweet little polio girl smile of glossed over gladness and carried on once more.

Mr. Curry said that transportation would be a life-long problem and as I prepared for the future, I needed to understand that. I told him I planned to drive. "Oh, no," he said. "I've seen people with more arm strength than you and they have been unable to drive. You might as well make up your mind to it. "Transportation will be a problem all of your life." He offered no solutions. He simply was bent on pointing out the difficulties that lay ahead of me. I continued to shut out his *not very helpful* observations, constantly reminding myself that I needed Mass Rehab to assist me and that man sitting across from me was trained by that commission to serve it–not me.

I was pleased that I did not need them for financial help initially at BU, since I received enough scholarship money for the first two years' tuition.

Tuition money was harder to come by later and Mass Rehab helped in my Junior and Senior years with both tuition and transportation costs.

But, Paul Curry was partially correct about transportation. It became a problem that needed to be solved every inch of the way. After graduating from BU, I took my first job as an elementary school counselor and teacher at St Pats, mainly because I needed the money to buy a car, not because I wanted the teaching job. I figured on working the job at St Pats Parochial School for two years and then moving on. What I hadn't counted on was liking the job, liking the kids so much and fending my way through it to a professional level which led to Graduate School and a Masters of Education in Counseling Degree.

I called Mass Rehab at that time for advice about auto hand controls and learning to drive. Maybe I wasn't clear about what I was asking, because all the counselor on the other end of the line said was that Mass Rehab didn't buy cars for clients. There was no advice offered about hand controls or learning to drive. So I turned to the Yellow Pages and found a car dealership that advertised "Hand Controls." I called Garber Auto School because they advertised instruction with hand controlled equipped cars. The instructor came out. I got behind the wheel and found I couldn't use their controls. They required strength different from mine. The instructor said I couldn't drive. I knew I couldn't drive with their controls. But I had come too far to quit and

174

couldn't let that stop me. I knew if I found the right controls I'd be able to drive, so I sent away for brochures on all the hand controls made everywhere on the planet. *"Gresham"* hand controls looked right at me, because they required the kind of strength I had.

Dad came through and did what I needed him to do. He took me to Arrow Pontiac in Arlington. I met the salesman, Hank Shomer, and told him I had exactly $2,500.00 and I described the car I needed. The car had to be just right for me and my wheelchair. I couldn't lift the chair in and out myself and would have to have someone put it in behind the front seat, so the door opening had to be wide enough for the chair to be moved in and out and for me to transfer my body easily into the chair. So a two door car with the wider door openings would be required. For the rest, I needed an automatic transmission, power steering and power brakes. That was it. No frills. Just car. Dad walked away and stared out the window the whole time I talked with Hank about it.

So almost ten years after my last conversation with Mr. Curry, I bought my first car–a 1967 Metallic Green Pontiac Tempest Coupe!!!

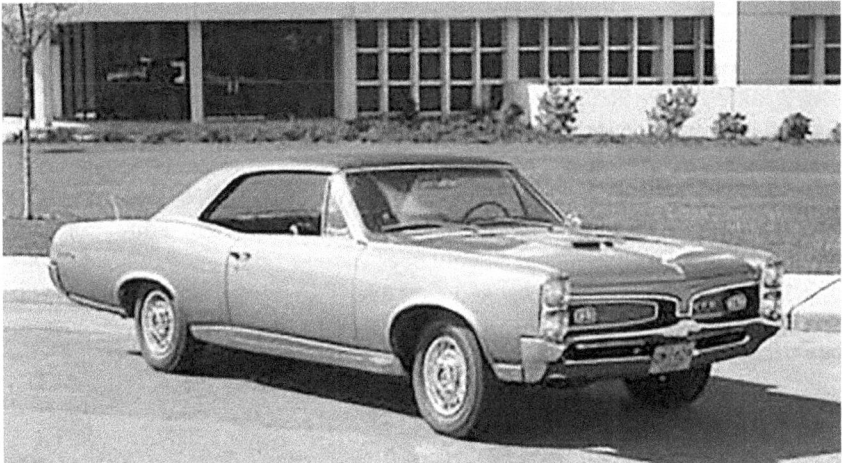

1967 Green Metallic Pontiac Tempest Coupe!!!

Dad and I picked it up at Arrow Pontiac on June 17, 1967.

He drove it home and parked it in the driveway. He had done just what I had asked him to do and he stayed very quiet. I had the Gresham car controls installed and found a driving instructor willing to teach me in my own car. Dad was very nervous about the whole thing. His nervousness matched my excitement. He was quiet, still and passive. I was full of fear but also super anxious to learn.

I found Mr. Taylor at the T&J Auto School of Winchester in the Yellow Pages. He was a tall, heavy set, friendly black man. He gave me ten road lessons during that cool and rainy summer. Mr. Taylor took a risk teaching me to drive because we had to use my car without dual controls for himself. He risked losing his license as an instructor. I was so grateful for his courage to deal with me. At first I had to have the hand controls adjusted to match my strength. Carroll Sleeper from Carlisle installed the controls. He worked on them until they were just right. Carroll was a disabled Vet and used hand controls himself. My left hand controlled the accelerator and the brake. My right hand controlled the steering with a spinning knob. He came to my house once a week and we went out on the road. In between, Dad, and sometimes Peggy went out with me.

In August, 1967 I got my license. I was thrilled and Mr. Taylor said "Now you can learn how to drive!" Dad's face almost fell off hearing that. He remained scared to death. So did Ma. They were happiest when the car was in the garage and I was in the house, but I went out anyway–always against their will. My teaching colleague and best friend, Ethel, was thrilled for me and very supportive. I had two trips I wanted to make right away. I wanted to go see Wini Wentworth Starbard in Holden. I got lost on the way and full of smiles, asked for directions at a gas station. I was thrilled to pieces when I pulled into Wini's driveway. My second trip was to Old Seabrook, Connecticut to see Mary Larange my best friend from High School. That was a long trip and I had to plan my rest stops. Mary gave me good directions and when I got there a cigarette and a cold beer were just the reward I needed. My metallic green Pontiac Tempest and every car I've owned since, has been my pride, joy, mobility and freedom. Especially my van. Since 1987 I've been able to use my electric wheelchair full time as a companion piece to my van. That meant and means even more independence and mobility.

Immediate solutions were not available in 1958 when Paul Curry had said that transportation would be a problem all of my life. Yes, it's expensive, it's a hassle and especially inconvenient when repairs are necessary, but it is wonderful! It has freed me from the bondage of yes, even Polio. It has been worth it all! It has been my delight. I sing praises every day with heartfelt grateful appreciation.

When I attended graduate school at Northeastern nights from 1967 until I got my Master's in 1971, I still used a manual wheelchair and I needed someone else to get the chair in and out of the car and I also needed someone to push me while I was out of doors. Frequently I drove to the Boston Campus in the late afternoon for a 4:15 class. I drove down Mass Ave past Symphony Hall and beyond Huntington Ave to take a right onto St. Botolph Street and drove past the old Industrial School for Crippled and Deformed Children–trying not to remember, but always did remember, as I pulled into the parking lot of the University. My left arm was just strong enough to make that journey in those early days. When there had been a lot of stopping and starting through traffic, my left arm and I barely made it into the parking space. One afternoon was especially scary. As I pulled into that familiar parking spot, the strength drained from my shoulder down through my elbow and wrist and drained out completely through my finger tips just as I came to a complete stop facing the gray stone building. Applying the hand brake with my left hand required every bit of strength that was left. I was shaking and exhausted as I rested my head on the steering wheel and breathed a prayer of gratitude and relief that I was safe.

Then, as always, I waited for someone to come along and help with the wheelchair. It was a nervous time–waiting, wondering if a friend would remember to meet me there before class. Usually, sure enough, someone would show up. My relief equaled the total draining of my physical energy. On those rare occasions when a friend would forget, I would hail a stranger passing by and bravely ask for help. Most people were gracious and eager to help and seemed glad to help. Others were reluctant and did help but only under some discomfort. I ignored their distress as I smiled and said "thanks." There was no other way. Amen, Lord, yes, Amen.

PART FOUR

My First Job

I ran into Father Smith after Sunday Mass in the Fall of 1963 and he asked me what I was doing now that I had graduated college. "Looking for a job," I said. Father Smith was the Pastor at St. Patrick's Parish and being the good friend that he was, he wanted me to have a job. He told me that he would ask Sister Gabriel, the Principal at St. Patrick's Grammar School, to think of a way to use me on their Staff. Shortly after, I received a call from Sister Gabriel asking me if I'd like to do some substitute teaching. And she said that she was also interested in hiring a Remedial Reading Teacher for the following academic year. There were twenty classrooms in 1964—grade One to Eight, around seven hundred kids. There were two classrooms for some grades and three for others. Sister Ann Cecelia was the Music Teacher and had the only extra available classroom.

Elementary Education had not occurred to me and returning to the Grammar School of my childhood was not the most attractive enticement beckoning me. But I needed to work and buying a car at the time was a clear-cut priority. I had the BA Degree and basically had decided to accept the 1st job that was offered, because I had already been interviewed several times without any other offers. Father Smith's offer was a "bird in the hand" so I took it. Harriet Rooney was teaching Fifth Grade and in the Spring of 1964 she agreed to have me do some observing and Student Teaching with her. I had known the School Nurse, Kay Kenny, years before. She had been the Public Health Nurse in the early days of my rehabilitation.

I enjoyed the classroom setting and getting to know the children. Since I had my Degree in English (Language and Literature) teaching Reading made some sense to me. I went back to B.U. during the Summer to the School of Education where Donald Durrell was Director of the Reading Clinic. I studied Methods of Teaching Reading and learned to administer Durrell's Analysis of Reading Difficulties. I learned what I needed to know to initiate a Remedial Reading Program at St. Patrick's in the Fall. I was paid $4,000.00 that first year. The Parish owned Kitty Lewis's little house on the corner of Pleasant and Central Streets, next to the newer of the two school buildings. It was used as the Religious Education, CCD (Confraternity of Christian Doctrine) Office, as well as the Parish Library. Pat McGah, the CCD Secretary, became a good friend along with the many women who volunteered for CCD, or in the Library. It was in that tiny building that I began the Remedial Reading Program. The house was not wheelchair accessible and Dad, who was driving me at the time, would bounce me up the steps into the building. There was no bathroom so I had to be sure I would not need to use a bathroom all day. My classroom stayed separated from the school for the first two years of my employment and I had little visual contact with the Faculty, or they with me. The Faculty Christmas Party was a dinner at The "Ship" Restaurant. No one had invited me to ride with them, but I was determined to join them, so I had Dad drive me there and pick me up. I had to count myself in because my being at the school as the Remedial Reading Teacher was not an Educational decision made by an eager Faculty. I was there because Sister Gabriel had created this job for me because Father Smith wanted me to have a job. I had established the Remedial Reading Program with little input from the other Teachers or from Sister Gabriel and felt that although the Faculty did cooperate with necessary things like fire drills and book donations, I needed to assert my individual place in their system, because beyond being an English Language and Literature Major, I valued the wonderfulness of Reading, had good organizational and interpersonal skills, a strong philosophy of learning, a strong belief in human potential and a strong desire to be there for the children. So I must say it was a successful venture for the children and for me. I found that on my own, I had the ability to design, implement and carry out a Remedial Reading Program, make a go of it and fit it into the fundamental goals of the school's overall educational framework.

At B.U. I had learned how to do a September Analysis of Reading Difficulties, prescribe a plan of remediation, teach in small groups, test, re-test and work closely with Teachers and Parents while the kids got the extra help with their Reading. The kids I dealt with were the little ones in First, Second and Third Grades. And there were the big kids in Sixth, Seventh, and Eighth Grades. Joanne O'Leary taught Seventh Grade and we became very good friends. Joanne encouraged me to go back to school for my Master's in Education. Joanne stood out from the rest of the Teachers. She was not entrenched or invested in Conservative Catholic thinking or in maintaining the status quo educationally. She did not see me as a Polio Victim given a job because Father Smith wanted it that way. Joanne recognized my strengths and professional capabilities. She was an intelligent, good natured and dynamic teacher who was always growing herself and she inspired growth in her students and in me. She challenged my thinking and professional methods. In the Fall of 1966 Sister Trinita became the new Principal. She was an awakened soul–interested and involved in life beyond the walls of our parochial elementary school and was willing to stretch and try new ways of teaching kids. She was supportive of me and the work I was doing. At Faculty meetings she would regularly ask for my point of view. Trinita saw what I was doing educationally and encouraged my full participation on the Faculty. I was validated as an Educator, Teacher, Counselor and most importantly as a Person.

After two years, Sister Ann Cecelia took her Music pupils over to the Convent on Pomworth Street where there were plenty of extra rooms and I moved into her old classroom in the newer of the two school buildings. I had earned my place in the scheme of things at St. Patrick's. Now I could be more visible and more readily available to the kids and the teachers.

The school building had one step that was never ramped during my tenure there and although there was an available bathroom I required assistance from the School Nurse who would open the door for me and stand outside to assure my privacy. It wasn't until 1973 that Congress passed The Rehabilitation Act that spoke to accessibility issues, mandating that schools and public buildings allow access for individuals with disabilities. After I left St. Patrick's, changes were made to accommodate BINGO players. The building got ramped and the bathroom was made accessible for all. Yeahhhhh! In 1966 Eighth Grade boys and girls were assigned to help me. They learned to get my manual wheelchair out of the car and position it for my transfer. They bounced me in and out of the building when I arrived in the morning and left in the afternoon. They also helped during Fire Drills. We became good buddies, learning to joke and be casual with each other. Some of those friendships remain today warming my heart with delight and appreciation. And 1966 was also a banner year for some new and permanent friendships–Connie Marquis, Irene Donovan, Sister Shawn and especially Ethel Choquette, who crashed into my world without any degree of pretention or mischief to become a lifelong motivator, supporter, protector and friend who also, along with the others, wanted to create a healthy academic environment for the children at St. Pats. She had arrived at St. Pat's in January, one month after she had left the convent in Florida where she had been a fully professed Sister of St. Joseph.

Ethel was bold and vigorous and had the courage of her convictions that buoyed us both up over the next few years. I was deeply insulated and far away and it took much boldness on her part to get me out of the house. At home the routine was firmly in place. Dad drove my car into the garage as soon as I got back from school in the mid-afternoon. He locked the garage door and parked his car in front of the door. I was tucked in for the night with Ma and Dad. Ma and Dad would say, "Watch out ! Be careful! Don't do that! Don't go there! Stay home! Don't get overtired. Don't get sick!" Old warnings from my early post-polio days never faded and came to be Ma and Dad's way

181

of keeping me close to home. Ethel's friendship became a threat to their tightly held world. "Don't trust her," Ma would say. But Ethel had crashed in and said "Come on! I want you to be my friend!" I was scared and excited at the same time. I didn't know what Ethel wanted. Ma kept telling me she was using me. Ma couldn't understand why she wanted me for her friend. She thought Ethel would find another friend–a boyfriend and drop me. Ma thought I'd get hurt. After I'd be out with Ethel, she would say "Thank you for being nice to Barbara." And Ethel would get furious and say "Mrs. Duffy, Barbara is my friend!" Ma just didn't understand that. She would lower her eyes and nod her head as if to say, "How nice of you–how kind." Ma just could never understand anyone choosing me for a friend. Neither could I, for that matter.

Yes, Ethel crashed on in and so did Irene. I noticed their spontaneity and enthusiasm and wanted to go along with them and I pushed hard against Ma and Dad and did go along with them. We all taught together at St. Pat's, so it wasn't as if I was a child then. Quite different. I was almost thirty. I had graduated from Boston University and was already working on my Master's Degree at Northeastern. I had developed the Remedial Reading program at St. Pat's and was teaching and consulting with parents and teachers. I'd taken my place in the professional community. But in my parent's eyes and at home I was still a child–the polio victim.

Infantilized, Paralyzed. When I pushed to be with Ethel and Irene Ma told me I was "a sap" for them. Especially if we used my car. Ma would say that Ethel and Irene were using me for my car. I didn't think so. And I wanted to go with them–to be with them. Even if they did use me for my car, I wanted to be with them. And so I did.

Ethel, Irene and I got our ears pierced!

Ethel pushed and pushed and pushed! She said, "You have to do this and this and that. If you want to be my friend you have to say "YES" when I ask you to do something!" Ethel and I went to the movies and to Hampton Beach where we put beach chairs on the sand and we sat on the beach for hours. I went everywhere Ethel went. I was scared but I liked it. Ma kept saying, "Don't trust her. She's French, She's crude. She's loud and noisy. She has poor taste. She doesn't dress nicely." And when Ethel met Phil, Ma said, "Ethel will drop you now that she has Phil." Phil pushed, too. He said, "You come, too." And I did. Ethel and Phil and I were together all the time. We went everywhere. We slept in a tent in the rain. We got wet. We fell down. And we laughed. We had long, long conversations. We stayed out very late at night. And when Ethel and Phil were planning their wedding Ethel wanted me to be her Maid of Honor, even though some of Ethel's relatives and friends thought like Ma and told Ethel not to have me in her wedding. Ma said Ethel was just making a show of herself, but Ethel said I was her best friend and she wanted me as her maid of Honor. I said, "Yes!" And on that day they gave me a gift that included these words:

"It is wrong to think that love comes from long companionship or persevering courtship. Love is the offspring of spiritual affinity and unless that affinity is created in a moment, it will not be created in years or even in generations." Kahlil Gibran

Working at St. Patrick's had given me the opportunity to pick up where I had left off when I was ten. Here I was at twenty-five, brought back to the very place I had been when Polio came along and provided that much needed detour. Now I could be with Sixth and Seventh and Eighth Graders and share their developmental experience. I saw myself in each one of them. Yes, I was there mainly to teach and guide them, yet in so doing I also allowed myself to work on my own pre-adolescent and adolescent psychosocial development that I had missed. The Seventh and Eighth Grade Girls would cram into my tiny classroom at lunch time to gossip about the boys, their families and themselves. We were doing parallel learning. Periodically, Trinita would scold all of us because her Rule was that *ALL* of the children should be outside of the building during Lunch Recess. The Education courses I was taking at Northeastern stimulated my interest in Curriculum Development and luckily by that time, along with Trinita, there were teachers on the Faculty who were also curious about creating a learning environment in which kids could learn, thrive and grow. The Faculty had grown. Those Faculty members treated me as a valued professional equal to themselves. We were of the mind that kids, like plants, would grow if we provided the right conditions and materials for their growth. If we provided the environment of support and encouragement and safety where risks could be taken, we would have a school without failure–where everyone grew at his/her own individual pace. Parents were involved in Parent Effectiveness Training and we Teachers as well took a course in Teacher Effectiveness Training. Vatican II had opened the window and let fresh air breathe upon re-examining Catholic ways of being in the world. The Liturgy was celebrated as a Folk Mass with exciting new music and Readings and Lay participation. Religious Education Conventions were dynamic, featuring the anti-war Berrigan Brothers (Daniel, a Jesuit Priest, and Peter, a priest of the Josephite order) and others who had the courage to embrace CHANGE and openly challenge the retrogressive Government policies.

From my perspective, I saw that healthy kids depended upon healthy families. Especially healthy mothers. In 1969-70, as I completed my Master

Barbara Lee Duffy & John M. Flynn

of Education in Counseling Degree, I offered a ten week group experience for mothers. Two hours on Thursday mornings became a time for mothers to focus, not on their kids, but on themselves. I taught the principals of Transactional Analysis and watched women come alive through both tears and laughter as they discovered and/or rediscovered their own thoughts, feelings and opinions. At the end of the year we had a Fun Day to celebrate and hug the five year old child within each of us and the mothers projected that joy onto their own offspring. The Mother's Group expanded to Tuesday mornings for new comers and continued on Thursday mornings for the on-going members. And eventually we had an evening group to include Dads. Every Spring we celebrated another Fun Day and once a year we traveled to the Weston Priory in Vermont to be uplifted and strengthened by the Benedictine Monks–their music and their living example of Peace, love and Justice.

More About St. Pats

The little children at St. Pat's were clear and spontaneous. They said what adults think, yet quickly suppressed it from themselves and from me. But they dared to look and ask, "Miss Duffy, what happened to your hand?" "Oh." And they would quickly draw away. I held my left hand in the strength of my right hand to tell them the story. "Yes, I know," I said. "It's weird looking at it for sure, isn't it–all the scars and stuff and those weird looking fingers, huh. I had a lot of operations on my hand to make it strong. Polio made my hand weak and the doctors made it strong again–strong enough to hold a pencil and pick up a book and strong enough to give hugs. And strong enough to use the hand controls in my car!" By that time they would be engaged and focused on the hand without feelings of disgust or anything like that and I would continue, "I think of that hand as my broken wing. It's precious to me because it has gone through so much and tries so hard and actually does so much for me every day. So now I put rings on my fingers and polish my nails and I take pride in the way my hand looks and is."

"Wow, Miss Duffy, I don't think your hand is weird. It's not funny looking. I think its fine. It's okay." A chorus of kid's voices agreed. "See, it's okay to come near to see and touch. And to get a warm hug."

Susan Bradford was in Sister Kathleen Marie's Homeroom. I saw Susan and a few other sixth graders for remedial reading and a counseling group. It was my time to do sixth grade for me, since that was when polio had stepped in and stole sixth grade away from me. I was almost thirty when I did that sixth grade class with Susan and Debbie and their friends.

Parallel learning! We had a pretty good time of it. I was "Miss Duffy" and the kids liked the time we spent together as much as I did.

One incident stands out in my mind. Behaving very unlike herself one afternoon, Susan sulked and pouted and slid down in her chair across from me. When I called attention to her she pulled herself up and out of herself with a start and assured me she was just fine. She stayed connected with my concern as she slid back down into herself, until I prodded enough and she said, "Miss Duffy, are you in pain all the time?" "You mean like when you kids give me a pain in the neck?" "No, no."

"Why do you ask Susan? What's going on?"

"Well, Miss Duffy," she said, "Sister was talking about you in class today. She said 'How many of you would like to be like Miss Duffy? She suffers all day, she has pain all day and she comes to work. How would you like to be like her?"

"Oh, my goodness, Susan. You know me so much better than Sister does."

"Do you suffer, Miss Duffy?"

"Oh, my dear Susan. Because I use a wheelchair, I am here with you now. I am here working at St. Pat's and while my friends from college are teaching and working in many other places, I am here now because I need to be here. I love you and I'm glad to be here. I have no physical pain. I'm sad sometimes because there are things I can't do. Things I'd like to do but can't. I've always loved the water and I think that if I could I would love to water ski. I can't and I'll never have a chance to try. And that makes me sad. When I was fourteen I cried and cried because I realized that I'd never walk in a pair of high heel shoes wearing a sexy stylish dress. That made me very sad. Now I know there are lots of wonderful things I can do. And being here with you is one of them. I love being a teacher. I love being with my friends. I love driving my car. I love to travel and study and learn new things. There are lots of things I love to do. And one of my favorite things is being here with you and Diane and Debbie and all the other kids."

Susan smiled. A few days later she said, "Well, Miss Duffy, Sister was talking about you again today and she said, 'Would any of you like to be like Miss Duffy?' I wanted to raise my hand and say yes, I'd like to be like Miss Duffy, but I didn't dare"

I was filled with warmth and love and appreciation for my young friend Susan–for my good fortune of being there and being available to hear and receive this gift of sheer joy.

In 1975 my work shifted and broadened beyond the Grammar School to serve the Parish as a whole. I retained the title of Teacher/Counselor and became a member of the Religious Education Team along with Father Jack Crowley, Maureen McMann and Sister Ann Carver. My work continued with the school kids and expanded to include Pre-Confirmation counseling for High School Students and Young Adult TA Growth Groups, development of Adult Religious Education events, as well as participation in the Pre-Marriage Program.

When I left St. Patrick's in 1979, I was forty years old and ready to take my place in the world. I had grown into a young adult. When I left

St. Patrick's I had a Master's Degree, fifteen years of experience and was earning $11,500.00.

I stood on a new and exciting threshold.

Transition

Jack Dyer taught Art at St. Pat's the first year I was there. He had blue, smiling Irish eyes and dark hair that was beginning to gray. We were friends and we have never lost contact. We haven't missed a Christmas greeting yet. Jack married and has one daughter, Erin. Jack left St. Pat's to be a Combat Artist for the Marine Corp in Viet Nam and he has worked at the Military Art Museum since that time. It was strange that Jack taught Art at St. Pat's and strange that we were friends. I liked Jack and he liked me. I liked his art work and he liked that I liked it. There was a gentle drawing together of the two of us. And a strange discomfort. I was twenty-five and still too shy to be sure of myself. I did feel Jack's presence. I felt his hands reach out toward me from behind as I sat at my teaching desk. I stayed very still. I felt his words in conversation, his smiling eyes–his gentle, deliberate hands. We spent much time together. We talked. I was still and distant. A few of us gathered in his apartment on the third floor of a house on Lindenwood Ave and he carried me up the flights of stairs.

I wanted a friendship with Jack. But I had no picture in my imagination of what an adult relationship with a man would look like. He slipped away. Yet Jack was the closest I ever came to having a boyfriend. But I had no pictures in my mind of me having a boyfriend or no mind pictures to verify even a possible boyfriend. I had no way of thinking about that. And no one else had a picture that might help either. When I tried to create pictures of an adult me, I had no pictures of me as a woman–as a sexual person, attractive and nice to be with. At that time, there was still nothing in my experience or frame of reference to support a picture of myself in a man-woman relationship. So I stayed child-like and withdrew from adult conversations about dating and boyfriends. That was out of sync for me. I felt inadequate and continued to mask it all with a polite shyness. It never occurred to me then that perhaps I was not attracted to men in a sexual way. And it never occurred to me that I could be attracted to women! Not even expectations that I would be sexual at all! I was after all, a sick child. Infantile paralysis had frozen me in at age ten.

Ma and Dad still hovered over me. I saw no other way.

There was a woman I met at Northeastern. She was a married mother of three young children. I felt a strange stirring inside of me and a desire to be with her. To spend time together and we did. I felt jealous of her husband and curious about her life, her friends and her activities. I had strange jealousy dreams of being excluded, left out. I never thought that she didn't know, but I did notice and wonder.

I drink my early morning coffee and remember, after so many pages, why I am here, doing this, writing this...

Yes indeed. I am working on the narrative of my third decade... The 1960's–searching, believing, as James P. Carse does, that understanding the narrative character of my life will lead to understanding its inherent mysticism. Especially since the level of mysticism in that narrative character of my life has always made sense to me. It is on the everyday level–on the level of interaction with my family and my peers that life has not made so much sense. I was the misfit– socially and emotionally immature. Shy, quiet. Not taking my place–educationally, or socially–sitting back, too scared to speak up. Not knowing what to say. Speaking out of step. Off the mark. To the left of center. Not reflecting the mainstream. Not hitting the mark. So for the most part I stayed quiet. Listening. Watching. Smiling. Feeling small. Inadequate. Not quite as good as... or as grown up as... or not as smart as... still a victim of infantile paralysis...

So much happened during the 60's to me, personally and to the world outside of me. The turbulent 60's! My third decade–the decade of my twenties. And although the days seemed to pass slowly and without fan-fare, the days were pregnant with new life teeming, in fact, with possibilities. Pathways deepened inward bringing me to a world beyond this world which would be my place of shelter and refuge and strength and replenishment on my journey. My monastery... because God was asking this of me. I am here today because I was there then.

Peggy and husband Paul and the three children lived around the corner since moving back to Stoneham from Georgia. Paul's job with General Electric had moved them from Boston to Schenectady, New York and back to Boston where John was born in 1959, then to Georgia for five years and the birth of Sharon in 1962, then back to Boston in 1965. In 1967 Peggy's family was becoming central to Ma and Dad's life and mine. They met at Starlight, the outdoor ballroom in Lynnfield. Peggy and Paul loved to dance. He was tall–6'2". They looked good together. Ma was pleased. And he was a Catholic! A strong believer!!!Peggy had lots and lots of boyfriends but Paul Murphy was always Ma's favorite.

Finally! Peggy had done something Ma could see and appreciate!

She produced beautiful, healthy, bright, babies! Ma couldn't get over it! She praised Peggy day in and day out for being so good with her babies! And Peggy loved her children. Ma said Peggy came by that naturally from Dad's side of the family. Dad loved kids. So did Aunt Dot and Aunt Nora. Not so much Dad's Ma—Ma Duffy. She was too busy dealing with her alcoholic husband and attending to her neighbors problems to have that much time for her own beyond dishing out stern directions.

Peggy and Paul were conscientious parents. No junk food! Brush those teeth! Peggy's full time job was taking care of the kids! And cooking! And she was a sterling cook! Ma glowed with pride over Peggy's cooking! And how well she set her table! Peggy shared her three kids with both Paul's and our families. She placed Susan on my lap saying, "Auntie Barb loves you!" For both the Murphys and the Duffys these were the only grandchildren. Peggy and Paul were the center of attention for holidays and birthdays and special occasions. We all took great pride in the three kids, Susan and John and Sharon.

Peggy's decision to divorce Paul took total courage as there was no support anywhere because Paul was loved and admired by everyone. I had a hard time testifying in court for Peggy, because I knew that Paul was not *cruel and abusive* in any physical way, but at the time they were going through the divorce, someone had to be the bad guy, because there were only a few legally acceptable reasons to obtain a divorce and one of the few was *cruel and abusive* behavior, so Paul had to be it. He and I talked and he said, "Look, Barb, I know. But we have to do it this way. It's okay. I understand."

Meanwhile brother Paul had become a stabilizing spiritual influence on the people of Taiwan, where he learned the language and discovered a brand new life of peace and fulfillment.

After their divorce, Paul Murphy went home to live with his parents, but he was never further away than the nearest telephone. He remained Peggy's best friend and stayed close to the kids. We all did. And Peg's love for the kids kept the channels open. Both families joined together on Christmas Eve, Thanksgiving and Easter and on each and every birthday. No one wanted the family to fall apart so no one missed a beat. Peggy flirted a bit with the town cops and flattered the local clergy. Other than that, she never entered into a serious, romantic relationship that I know of...

In 1990 Paul Murphy married Nancy. They have a nice home and they visit the homes of the kids at least twice each year.

After Ma died, Peggy walked around the house and removed all the pictures of her children and her grandchildren. As if speaking only to herself, she moved methodically from photo to photo, taking each one in both of her hands saying, "This is mine, this is mine and this and this" until every picture was gone. I watched with great sadness... but I thought of this narrative right here and how my memories continue to flow openly and truthfully on this parchment–I have the comforting knowledge that this story–my story, is a story no one can steal. I and my soul mate Jackie Flynn will make sure of that.

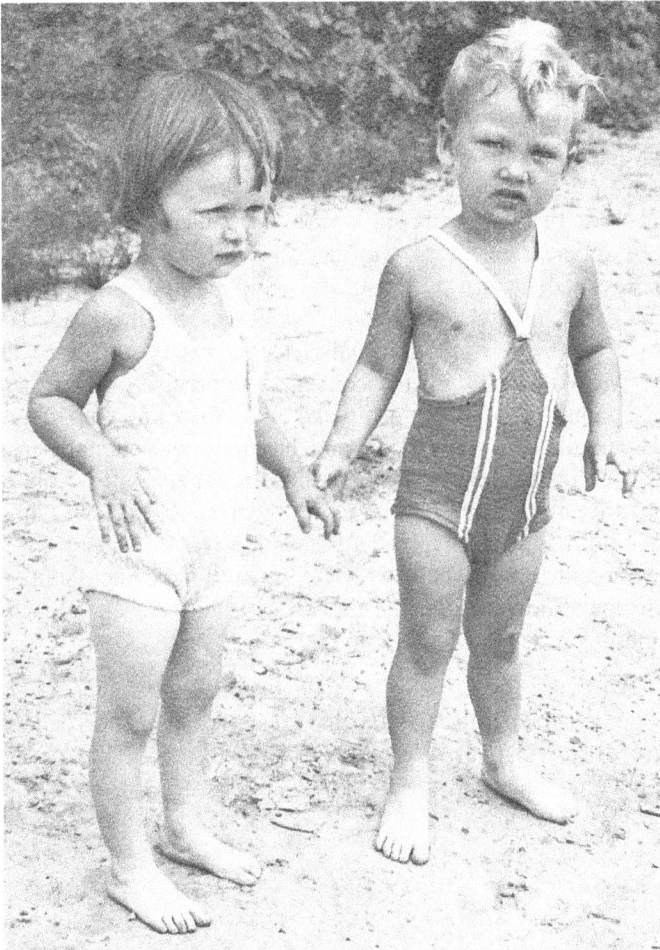

Barbara Duffy & Jackie Flynn–Soul-mates since birth, in 1939.

Jackie

In the fifties, I read Jack Kerouac's *On The Road* and *The Subterraneans*. I was fifteen when I read Huxley's Brave New World and reread it again and again, and Whitman's *Song of Myself*. And I was twenty when cousin Jackie walked out of Salem State Teachers college after his sophomore year and with a copy of *On the Road* in his pocket he hitched a ride on a cross-country rig, first to Juarez, Mexico, then to L.A. and Venice California, then up the coast to San Francisco. I would have traveled with him that summer... if my life had been different... if polio had not claimed me as her own. As it was, I did travel with him, vicariously, never really knowing the depth of his experiences out there. We stayed connected by letters and his infrequent visits during the next ten years. Those years took Jackie far away into the world of psychedelic drugs, mysticism, Sufism and Yoga in search of himself. During those ten years that Jackie was on the road, I felt that I was traveling with him, spiritually. Every two years or so he would return and we would pick up the conversation precisely where we had left off. It was so comforting–the kinship and unspoken knowing between us– the mutual anguish, smiles of joy and harmony–our eternally inseparable two lives. Jackie's life experience was my intimate, soulful connection to one's outward journey in search of my own soul, as I was his link to one's inner journey. I was forced to stay. He was forced to go. We visit together now and return where we were so long ago. Each supporting the other with unconditional love–the mutual gift we have given each other in this lifetime.

Neither of us could help it. Our destinations–our destinies were directed by the whispering spirit behind each of us. The roads we have taken were different roads, but the right road for each, and the only road we could have taken.

To Live, To Care, To Love

As I sit down again, on a seemingly average day, to write more of Miss Duffy's great life adventure and personal philosophy, I realize on this day, that it can no longer be simply an objective observational vantage point for the purpose of examination and explication anymore, for my mind is preoccupied–distracted.

You see, Joey was twelve years old–a seventh grader at my school. He underwent corrective heart surgery yesterday and died on the operating table. How can I go in there and face the other children–especially Michael. He was Joey's best buddy. Joey was so bouncy and bright eyed last week and we all looked forward to his surgery which would correct his congenital heart defect. Today we did not speak of details. I don't know what went wrong. All I know is Joey didn't make it. A child asked, "Why did Joey die Miss Duffy?" looking at me with full eyes, expecting so, so much. What could I say to that child? I didn't know why Joey died any more than he did. My mind became absorbed in reflection–eternal reflection. That day, changed everything again.

6 months later...

I was talking with a seventh grade boy today and I asked him what he wanted to be when he grew up. He thought awhile and said, "Miss Duffy, one day Monsignor put his hand on my head and said, 'You have the head of a Bishop,' so I guess I'll be a Bishop." Then I said, "And if you don't become a Bishop, what would you like to be?" And he replied, "A baseball player!"

There is still sorrow in me these days because of Joey and still a few misunderstandings between and among some family members. And pain within me because of some friendships that have left scars based on old, erroneous judgments and threatened values of one sort or another. Many of them half-forgotten and/or impossible to mend because the person or persons have moved or passed away.

And yet deep within me there is tranquility, peace, joy and love that find no words, but flowing through my being, celebrating life, there is meaning and direction that transcends the activity of my daily life. The sorrow, the pain, the occasional loneliness is acute. But not without purpose. Not without growth. Not without continuing creativity. And now and then the silence within me speaks to the silence within another and I give thanks for a new day of loving. The continual seeking, the crying in the night, the oft repeated leaning over the abyss gives birth to new life within me.

Mary and I

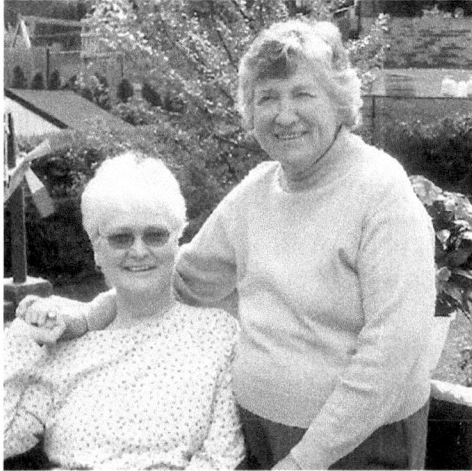

Barbara Mary

At this time of my life I couldn't be happier. My dear friend and love of my life, Mary Armato and I are basking in the sunshine at the Visitor's Center of the Western Priory in Western, Vermont. We are here together, loving deep into the gift of our faith, friendship and mutual devotion–rising early to be here and ready to join with our brothers and sisters to pray, sing, break bread and be one with all there is. Oh such brilliance! Nothing more to ask for in this whole wide world. A sense of deep joy, bathed in sunlight on a Saturday morning.

"Why, who makes much of a miracle?

As to me,

I know of nothing else but Miracles..."

Walt Whitman

Epilogue

I awake at dawn and give thanks for another day. I rise and come to my writing table to sing praise–to rejoice–to grieve–to weep–to speak words of love and words of despair. *A Winter's Solstice* plays softly in the background. The haunting sounds of the flute–the grounding tones of the piano. Outside my window the wind blows the winter's cold, yet I am warm and snug. Even my toes are warm. I wait and recall forgotten times. I draw upon a memory to put together a memoir. A hymn. A song. Bringing me back to the God within–the Goddess within, whom I have found and have loved all these days. The sleet hits against my window. Cars begin to rush by... Bless this work I do, Lord, bless this early morning rising.

I am holding the residue of all that has preceded this moment. I am holding all that I have become. I will defend my life. This is my right and my obligation. This is who I am and how I want to be... and what have I found...

Silence–deep penetrating, wordless silence!

www.ingramcontent.com/pod-product-compliance
Lightning Source LLC
Chambersburg PA
CBHW062054270326
41931CB00013B/3076